Practical Procedures in Dental Occlusion

To my 2Ms: my wife Manal and son in law Mohsi
To my 3Ls: my daughters Loujin, Lilas and Leanne

Ziad Al-Ani

To the Creator, My Mother and Father, Wife Azmat and my 4 children Zayd, Adam, Esa, Khadijah

Riaz Yar

Practical Procedures in Dental Occlusion

Ziad Al-Ani, BDS, Oral Surg PG Dip, Fixed Pros PG Dip, PGCAP, MSc, PhD, MFDS RCS(Ed), FHEA, RET Fellow
Senior Lecturer
School of Medicine, Dentistry & Nursing
University of Glasgow, UK

Riaz Yar, BDS, MFDS RCS (Edin), MPhil (Restorative), DPDS, Dip Implant Dent RCS (Edin), MPros Dent RCS (Edin), FDS RCS (Edin), Masters in Soft Tissue around Teeth and Implants (Bologna)
Director and Visiting Professor
The Square Advanced Dental Care
Hale Barns, UK

WILEY Blackwell

Registered Offices
John Wiley & Sons, Inc., 111 River Street, Hoboken, NJ 07030, USA
John Wiley & Sons Ltd, The Atrium, Southern Gate, Chichester, West Sussex, PO19 8SQ, UK

Editorial Office
9600 Garsington Road, Oxford, OX4 2DQ, UK

For details of our global editorial offices, customer services, and more information about Wiley products visit us at www.wiley.com.

Wiley also publishes its books in a variety of electronic formats and by print-on-demand. Some content that appears in standard print versions of this book may not be available in other formats.

Library of Congress Cataloging-in-Publication Data

Names: Al-Ani, M. Ziad, author. | Yar, Riaz, author.
Title: Practical procedures in dental occlusion / Ziad Al-Ani, Riaz Yar.
Description: First edition. | Hoboken, NJ : John Wiley & Sons, 2022. |
       Includes bibliographical references and index.
Identifiers: LCCN 2021013458 (print) | LCCN 2021013459 (ebook) | ISBN
     9781119678519 (paperback) | ISBN 9781119678489 (adobe pdf) | ISBN
     9781119678526 (epub)
Subjects: MESH: Dental Occlusion | Malocclusion–prevention & control |
     Orthodontics, Corrective–methods
Classification: LCC RK523 (print) | LCC RK523 (ebook) | NLM WU 440 | DDC
     617.6/43–dc23
LC record available at https://lccn.loc.gov/2021013458
LC ebook record available at https://lccn.loc.gov/2021013459

Cover Design: Wiley
Cover Image: © Ziad Al-Ani

Set in 9.5/12.5pt STIXTwoText by Straive, Pondicherry, India
Printed and bound by CPI Group (UK) Ltd, Croydon, CR0 4YY

C9781119678519_201223

Contents

Acknowledgements

The authors wish to acknowledge the kind permission of Claire O'Connor, Neil Sparkes and Deborah Khadem in using them as photographic models in some chapters of this book.

We are very grateful to Tanya McMullin, Loan Nguyen and Bhavya Boopathi for their advice and support in the production of this text.

We would like to thank Mr Robert Gandy, Ceramist, The Cube Advanced Dental Laboratory for the Wax up on the front page and all the ceramic restorations documented in the book.

About the Companion Website

Don't forget to visit the companion website for this book:

www.wiley.com/go/al-ani-and-riaz/dental-occlusion

There you will find valuable material designed to enhance your learning, including:

- Videos
- Figures from the book as downloadable PowerPoint slides

About the Book

The subject of occlusion has traditionally been very difficult to learn, understand and manage. As a result, an unwanted mystique has been built around it that has intimidated a large part of the dental profession.

It is now more important than ever that dental practitioners familiarise themselves with a subject that so intimately affects their daily professional lives.

Restorative treatment outcome is highly dependent on the occlusion of the restoration when the treatment is complete and therefore sound up-to-date knowledge of all evidence-based aspects of this commonly encountered condition is essential.

General practitioners usually have very limited practical clinical experience in occlusion and most of the books available for them are theory-based resources.

This book aims to enable readers to gain a solid foundation of knowledge of occlusion, by providing practical, learnable, usable information and techniques which are demonstrated in a practical and easy-to-understand style. The intention is to explain current evidence-based practical concepts in the field of dental occlusion so that they can be reflected in the reader's clinical practice.

The book contains a series of everyday clinical situations in occlusion, that may be encountered in general practice, to help readers understand and engage with the information and to promote effective clinical management.

It aims to provide practical guidance to what is required to optimise restorative treatment outcomes, including occlusion, in simple and advanced restorative care. The book also promotes learning as a dynamic process of active involvement. It encourages valuation by self-assessment with questions at the end of the book.

Chapter 1 – Terminology

It is important we address terminology right at the start to reduce the confusion that has been created throughout the history of occlusion. As a source, Glossary of Prosthodontic Terms 2017 edition is used throughout the book.

Chapter 2 – Neuroanatomy – Why is It Important?

This chapter will address neuromuscular philosophies and introduce the neurolink between all systems from the periodontal mechanoreceptors on teeth through to central pattern generators in the pons and muscles and temporomandibular harmony.

Chapter 3 – What's of Use to Me in Practice? Armamentarium, Equipment and Techniques

This is a 'how-to' chapter. It is important for the clinician to know the equipment and techniques used in occlusal examination, registration and record. This chapter also discusses facebow, articulators and how to make a stabilisation splint.

Chapter 4 – I Don't Know What I Am Recording Where are the True Contacts?

This chapter illustrates a classic problem most of the practitioners face when recording occlusal contacts using different articulating papers. It will highlight the following:

- morphology and type of occlusal contacts in class 1, class 2 and class 3 relationships
- the importance of selecting the correct size of articulating papers
- the appropriate techniques in recording occlusal contacts
- how to properly mark shiny occlusal surfaces.

Chapter 5 – The Crown is High

This clinical scenario will highlight the possible factors which may contribute to this situation (a high crown). It discussed the importance of accurate opposing alginate impression and mounting of the casts. The laboratory handling of the cast and the provisional crown will be covered.

Chapter 6 – My Bite Feels Different

Using a clinical scenario of a change of patient bite following fitting of an indirect restoration, this chapter will mainly focus on the importance of adopting the conformative approach in restorative dentistry. The possibility of introducing iatrogenic changes to a patient's bite is quite real and can have immediate consequences. Avoidance of the problem is the best approach but to do this, you must be aware of the potential pitfalls in restorative care.

Chapter 7 – My Front Tooth Filling Keeps Fracturing

This clinical scenario of a fractured upper central incisor composite restoration will highlight the importance of checking premature contacts in centric relation and dynamic occlusion.

Chapter 8 – TMD and Occlusion – Is There a Link?

Opinion regarding the importance of occlusion as an aetiological factor in the development of TMDs has shifted between it being the main causative factor and there being no correlation at all. This chapter will discuss this controversy and provides the reader with findings from contemporary literature.

Chapter 9 – How Would I Adjust a High Occlusal Contact?

This chapter will explain the proper techniques which should be adopted when adjusting the occlusal contacts and interferences by the dentist.

Chapter 10 – How Would I Ensure a Good Occlusion on Posterior Composite Restorations?

This chapter will illustrate the concepts and practical steps of achieving occlusal surfaces which provide proper reconstruction of natural morphology. It will highlight the following aspects:

- conforming to existing guidance in restored teeth
- creating departure clearance spaces
- the importance of the location of the occlusal contact.

Chapter 11 – My Front Teeth Feel Loose and Are Moving

This chapter will discuss occlusal trauma from functional or parafunctional forces. Lack of freedom in centric and the effect of RCP–ICP slide on anterior teeth will be also covered.

Chapter 12 – Canine Guidance or Group Function?

This has been an ongoing debate over many years with discussions on which lateral-based occlusal scheme is the best for the patient. This chapter will discuss the rationale behind both and how to achieve them clinically.

Chapter 13 – Replacing Missing Teeth – Abutment is Involved with Guidance

This clinical scenario will highlight the flowing points:

- checking the guidance prior to commencing treatment
- conforming to the guidance by selecting a treatment plan which avoids changing it.

Chapter 14 – The Space is Lost! Loss of Occlusal Space Following Crown Prep

This chapter will discuss the significant concepts which need to be understood and planned when considering restoration of a tooth involved in the centric relation/retruded contact position. How to manage when the space is suddenly lost during crown preparation on a tooth that is the last in the arch.

Chapter 15 – My Front Teeth Are Worn

Management of tooth surface loss is a complex treatment but some straightforward rules will help in diagnosis of the cause, monitoring of the situation and its management.

This chapter will illustrate the principles of management of non-carious tooth surface loss (TSL) cases and will focus on:

- achieving an appropriate OVD (when and how)
- review of mounted study casts
- diagnostic wax-up
- Dahl concept.

Chapter 16 – All My Teeth Are Restored But Don't Meet Like They Did Before

In this chapter, a patient has presented with a restored mouth with multiple crowns and they feel the teeth do not meet like before. They cannot find a comfortable position. The use of material that allows testing the increase of OVD when managing advanced restorative care cases will be discussed. A full description of clinical procedure will be offered here.

Chapter 17 – I Am Breaking My Teeth and Veneers and Lost a Tooth Due To Grinding

The following points are discussed in this chapter:

- OVD increase
- improving incisal and occlusal relationships
- rule of thirds
- aesthetic and functional analysis.

Chapter 18 – Occlusion on Implants. Any difference?

Dental implants may be more prone to occlusal overloading. A primary cause of peri-implantitis and bone loss around implants is the excessive force applied from unwanted occlusal contact. The occlusal prescription of an implant-supported restoration, therefore, has to be much more carefully designed than that on a natural tooth. The 10 principles of occlusion over implants are discussed in this chapter.

Glossary of Terms

This is more of a dictionary of terms than merely a glossary of terms used in this book. This chapter isolates the relevant terms from the glossary of prosthodontic terms. published regularly in the Journal of Prosthetic Dentistry.

Short Answer Questions

This chapter includes short answer questions for the reader to practise. The knowledge gained from reading this book will enable the reader to answer these questions effectively.

1

Terminology

It is important we address terminology right at the start to reduce the confusion that has been created throughout the history of occlusion. As a source, we will use the Glossary of Prosthodontic Terms (GTP) (2017) edition for the most part.

The three most important terms are defined below.

Centric occlusion (CO) – the occlusion of opposing teeth when the mandible is in centric relation (CR); this may or may not coincide with the maximal intercuspal position (MICP) (GTP 2017). Throughout the literature (Jiménez-Silva et al. 2017, McNamara et al. 1995, Shildkraut et al. 1994, Weffort and de Fantini 2010), centric occlusion is also known as intercuspal or MICP and hence the confusion because the same term can indicate two different positions. So, to prevent further confusion, we will state that centric occlusion is MICP.

Centric relation – this position has five main points:

1) a maxillomandibular relationship, independent of tooth contact
2) the condyles articulate in the anterior–superior position against the posterior slopes of the articular eminences
3) the mandible is restricted to a purely rotary movement
4) from this unstrained, physiological, maxillomandibular relationship, the patient can make vertical, lateral, or protrusive movements
5) it is a clinically useful, repeatable reference position.

Each statement can be debated and to achieve consensus may be difficult, but the key point is that this is a tooth-independent position, i.e. it can be recorded in edentulous patients. We feel that first statement is incomplete, and would add: a maxillomandibular relationship, independent of tooth contact at the correct occlusal vertical dimension (OVD) for that individual.

Centric relation contact position (CRCP) – the occlusion of opposing teeth when the mandible is in centric relation; this may or may not coincide with the MICP (GTP 2017). This may involve one pair of teeth or several pairs or may coincide with all the teeth meeting. When the teeth touch then they slide from that position into MICP. According to Posselt (1952), 90% of the population have a discrepancy between both positions.

Practical Procedures in Dental Occlusion, First Edition. Ziad Al-Ani and Riaz Yar.
© 2022 John Wiley & Sons Ltd. Published 2022 by John Wiley & Sons Ltd.
Companion website: www.wiley.com/go/al-ani-and-riaz/dental-occlusion

Other important terms are given in the table below and will be defined throughout the book and in the Glossary.

Term	Other names in the literature	Terms we will use in the book
Centric occlusion	Maximal intercuspal position, intercuspal position	Centric occlusion (CO)/intercuspal position (ICP)/maximal intercuspal position (MICP)
Centric relation	Terminal hinge axis or retruded axis position	Centric relation (CR)
Centric relation contact position (CRCP)	Retruded contact position, centric occlusion	Centric relation contact position (CRCP)
Maximal intercuspal position	Centric occlusion, intercuspal position, habitual occlusion, bite of convenience	Centric occlusion (CO)/intercuspal position (ICP)
Occlusal vertical dimension (OVD)	Vertical dimension of occlusion (VDO), dimension of vertical occlusion (DVO)	Occlusal vertical dimension (OVD)
Rest vertical dimension (RVD)	Rest position, physiological rest position, vertical dimension of rest	Rest vertical dimension (RVD)
Freeway space	Interocclusal distance	Interocclusal distance
Bennett angle	Progressive side shift	Bennett angle
Bennett shift (movement)	Immediate side shift	Bennett shift (movement)
Working side movement	Laterotrusive, laterotrusion	Working side movement
Non-working side movement	Mediotrusive, Mediotrusion	Non-working side movement

References

(2017). The Glossary of Prosthodontic Terms: ninth edition. *J. Prosthet. Dent.* 117: e1–e105.

Jiménez-Silva, A., Tobar-Reyes, J., Vivanco-Coke, S. et al. (2017). Centric relation–intercuspal position discrepancy and its relationship with temporomandibular disorders. A systematic review. *Acta Odontol. Scand.* 75 (7): 463–474.

McNamara, J.A., Seligman, D.A., and Okeson, J.P. (1995). Occlusion, orthodontic treatment, and temporomandibular disorders: a review. *J. Orofac. Pain* 9: 73–90.

Posselt, U. (1952). Studies in the mobility of the human mandible. *Acta Odontol. Scand.* 10 (Suppl 10): 19–160.

Shildkraut, M., Wood, D.P., and Hunter, W.S. (1994). The CR-CO discrepancy and its effect on cephalometric measurements. *Angle Orthod.* 64: 333–342.

Weffort, S.Y.K. and de Fantini, S.M. (2010). Condylar displacement between centric relation and maximum intercuspation in symptomatic and asymptomatic individuals. *Angle Orthod.* 80: 835–842.

2

Neuroanatomy – Why is It Important?

Introduction

What is the role of the teeth? An important question which underpins our clinical dentistry because we are routinely involved in possibly changing it if we don't follow a careful process. The roles of the teeth can be thought of as follows.

- Mastication.
- Swallowing.
- Speech/phonetics.

This is a simplified view because the impact of teeth is far greater for both the individual but also when interacting with the wider community.

- Aesthetics – emotional and psychosocial perspective; this is specific to the individual and also has an impact on their self-esteem.
- Psychophysical – the ability to appreciate the food via texture, volume and taste.
- Occlusal stability and jaw support – maintain the elements that maximise function.
- Cognition – decreased mastication is a risk factor for dementia.
- Mortality – Osterberg et al. 2008 in numerous studies demonstrate the statistically significant correlation between the number of teeth remaining and mortality, with the data suggesting a 4% decrease in mortality for each remaining tooth above 20 occluding pairs. I am not suggesting that we tell our patients they will live longer if we provide more teeth but the link between quality of life and having fixed teeth is certain.

So how do we avoid altering this system in an uncontrollable manner? We use protocols and processes. The acronym for the process is STOP! STOP picking up that drill before you assess the occlusion. A preassessment of the occlusion is crucial to ensure we have not potentially affected the role or performance of the teeth. Therefore, we use our senses to preassess the occlusion. This is essential in both conformative and reorganised occlusion.

S – Survey – visual assessment using coloured paper to analyse contacts.
T – Touch – fremitus.
O – Observe and listen.
P – Patient feedback.

Practical Procedures in Dental Occlusion, First Edition. Ziad Al-Ani and Riaz Yar.
© 2022 John Wiley & Sons Ltd. Published 2022 by John Wiley & Sons Ltd.
Companion website: www.wiley.com/go/al-ani-and-riaz/dental-occlusion

The goals of occlusion are as follow.

- To provide equal contacts on as many teeth as possible when the patient swallows – centric occlusion position. This will aid muscle health.
- To provide incisional guidance (protrusive guidance) on the anterior teeth. This will aid temporomandibular joint health.
- To provide group function when chewing using cuspal inclines.
- To avoid introducing new contacts (unless in a controlled manner) which may strain the adaptive capacity of the patient.
- To biomechanically distribute the forces so as not to cause failure of the restoration or other teeth.

Neuroanatomy

The aim of this chapter is to provide a clear understanding of the complex neural framework involved in mastication, swallowing and speech. The key objective is the information the brain requires to understand the position of the jaw in space and it acquires this information from the teeth, temporomandibular joint (TMJ), muscles and soft tissues.

An understanding of the neural framework involved in dental occlusion is essential in determining the protocols within clinical dentistry. The neural framework comprises the central nervous system (CNS) (spinal cord and brain) and the peripheral nervous system (connects the rest of the body to the spinal cord and brain). This is a feedback and feedforward system made up of sensory fibres (registering pain, pressure and temperature) and motor fibres (providing a function such as muscle contraction).

Anatomically, another structure which is important in our understanding of the masticatory system is the brainstem, which is the posterior part of the brain continuous with the spinal cord which is composed of three regions:

- medulla oblongata
- pons
- mesencephalic area.

Why do I need to know this, I hear you ask? Well, within this area are the central pattern generators (CPGs) generally defined as a network of neurons (nerve cells) capable of enabling the production of central commands, specifically controlling stereotyped rhythmic motor behaviours such as mastication, deglutition, respiration and locomotion, among others. There is increasing evidence suggesting that some of these CPGs are interconnected for co-ordinated control.

In this chapter we will only be dealing with mastication and deglutition. For further reading, the article by Steuer and Guertin (2019) goes into greater detail. Kandel (2012) stated that the brainstem is an important element of motor and sensory function and plays a key role in the control of mastication and deglutition.

Mastication

This process needs sensory input for the CPGs and this comes from the periodontal mechanoreceptors (PDMRs), muscles, bones, TMJ and soft tissues. Other inputs from the higher centres of the brain can also affect the basic output from the CPG. The output through the motor fibres is relayed in the descending pathway to the muscles to apply forces to break food down. This process is constant and if we bite on something hard which we are not expecting then a reflex arc is created, i.e. jaw opening reflex (Figure 2.1).

Most foods that we are used to eating do not require attention, but when we try a new food the higher order brain centres are involved as we investigate (attention is required) this new substance in regard to texture and taste and a decision is made whether we will eat this again. This is feedforward learning. Age and types of food can also modulate mastication activity as stated by Peyron et al. (2004).

What is the Goal of Mastication?

The goal of mastication is to increase the surface area of food to enhance enzymatic action. Therefore, our teeth (incisors, canines, premolars and molars) are designed to crush and shear the food.

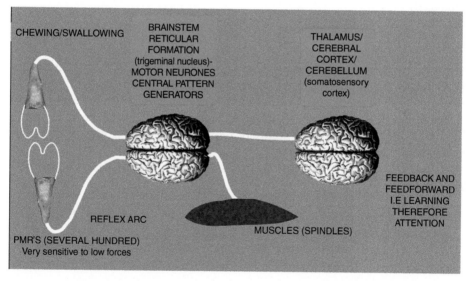

Figure 2.1 Signal pathways. PDMR (afferent neurons) are triggered (sensory and motor) and the impulse is detected in the trigeminal ganglion and the trigeminal mesencephalic nucleus. The information is then relayed at the brainstem and finally projected to the primary somatosensory cortex. The output from the cortex seems to be important for initiating and co-ordinating masticatory movement and adapting to the hardness of the bolus. *Source:* Modified from Morquette et al. (2012).

- Incisors – designed to grab and cut through food (to incise).
- Canines – designed to grab and tear through food (cornerstone of the arch).
- Premolars – designed to crush food and seen as transitional due to having anatomical features of both canines and molars (the equilibrium point of the arch).
- Molars – designed for grinding food.

The muscles involved in mastication are responsible for moving the jaws in a manner that brings the teeth into contact rhythmically. When the muscles are inflamed this process can be painful and uncomfortable. Certain activities can cause this such as:

- hypernormal function – habits such as nail biting, chewing gum
- parafunction – clenching (static) and bruxism (dynamic).

Muscles involved in jaw opening (smaller muscle mass group).

- Lateral pterygoid.
- Suprahyoid muscles – anterior digastric, mylohyoid, geniohyoid.

Muscles involved in jaw closing (larger muscle mass group underlying where the greater activity is).

- Temporalis.
- Masseter.
- Medial pterygoid

The innervation for these muscles is via the trigeminal nerve (V) but other cranial nerves such as the facial (VII), glossopharyngeal (IX) and hypoglossal (XII) are also involved in the whole process of mastication and swallowing, which comprises more than 30 nerves and muscles (Matsuo and Palmer 2008). Some of these muscles are also involved in respiration and are considered accessory respiratory muscles as discussed by Van Lunteren and Dick (1997).

The pattern of mastication is made up of three successive cycles as described by Lund (1991).

1) The *preparatory phase* – also called the gathering stage, when the incisors bring the food into the mouth and shift it deeper onto the posterior teeth.
2) The *reduction phase* – breakdown of food in a rhythm called the chewing cycle; as the food gets smaller, the teeth start to contact, letting us know that the food is ready for swallowing
3) The *preswallowing phase* – the bolus is prepared for swallowing, the tongue places the food posteriorly and the swallowing reflex is initiated.

The evidence also supports sensory feedback controls for a large part of the masticatory process. Soft foods mean a short masticatory sequence and tough foods provoke a longer sequence, as discussed by Plesh (1986).

Let's look at the sensory feedback system in more detail (Figure 2.2).

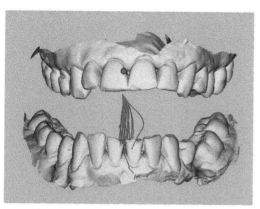
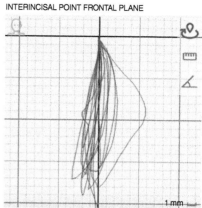

INTERINCISAL POINT FRONTAL PLANE

1 mm

Figure 2.2   Chewing cycle data collected using MODJAW (for further details on MODJAW see Chapter 12).

Sensory and Motor Feedbacks

PDMRs

Situated close to the collagen fibres and in between like a sandwich within the periodontal ligament and described as Ruffini-like by Byers (1985) and Lambrichts (1992) in humans. The main periodontal Ruffini nerve endings have been classified as type 1 and 2. Type 1 shows lamellar terminal Schwann cells and expanded axon terminals with axonal spines which penetrate surrounding tissue; type 2 is characterised by lesser branched Ruffini endings with fewer axonal spines, less basal lamina and fewer Schwann cells. Both of these receptor types are present in the periodontal ligament (Maeda et al. 1999).

These are crucial for force interpretation and control of mastication and therefore it would be assumed that the different teeth (incisors–molars) would have differing sensitivity thresholds and this has been shown to be correct by Johnsen et al. (2007). This is called the interocclusal tactility threshold (ITT) as discussed by Herren (1988) and this study uses foils of varying thickness between healthy teeth. The smallest ITT recorded is between 8 and 60 µm but during chewing the threshold increases by a factor of 5 (range 2.5–8×) and the occlusal perception is reduced due to descending inhibition (sensory gating), meaning there is a filtering out of irrelevant information which allows for enhanced detection of unexpected stimuli. There are also interindividual variations which are ascribed to differing attentional degrees in the higher brain centres and this will be linked to adaptability and neuroplasticity (capability to change and adapt to new demands).

The direction of force also shows that the PDMRs respond more when the forces are axial, i.e. in the direction in which they function best – 'Directional bias may reflect functional adaptation' (Sato 1988). When force is applied, the collagen fibrils are compressed which fires the mechanoreceptors. The use of the split and hold tests by Trulsson and Johansson (1996) also determined the amount of force required through a positive feedback loop, meaning the harder the food, the more force is applied through the initial feedback from the mechanoreceptors. A recent systematic review by Piancino et al. (2017) summarises studies that looked at this in greater detail.

What happens, then, when we lose teeth and the PDMRs are lost? Several studies such as Svensson and Trulsson (2011) and Svensson et al. (2013) have shown higher biting and food holding forces, indicating that optimal restoration design is fundamental.

Pulp

The pulp also provides proprioception. Randow and Glanz (1986) showed that non-vital teeth had mean pain threshold levels that, on cantilever loading, were more than twice as high as those of neighbouring or contralateral vital teeth. This partly explains the vulnerability to fracture of root-filled teeth.

Muscles

The control of position and movement of the muscle/tendon complex is achieved by a combined Golgi tendon organ (GTO) and muscle spindle (MS) feedback. The jaw closing muscles are richly supplied with MSs which provide information related to length and contraction velocity of muscle fibres and generate muscle activation patterns in a predictable manner. The GTO provides information related to tension of the tendons (Kistemaker et al. 2013). This is a feedback loop system which plays a role in CPGs and given the superior tactile discriminative abilities of dentate subjects in comparison with those with implant-supported or removable prostheses, PDMRs provide a more sensitive indicator of jaw position and movement.

What happens when we increase the occlusal vertical dimension (OVD)? An increase in OVD results in stretching or increased MS length. Muscles show a high degree of functional adaptability/plasticity; Yabushita et al. (2006) found that there is a significant decrease in MS sensitivity up to 2 weeks post increase of OVD. This has similarities to Clark et al.'s (1999) 68-year review on occlusal interference studies in that any muscle symptoms were transient. The changes in spindle function may be due to changes in occlusal function producing alterations in CNS masticatory controls combined with the different PDMR input. Therefore, to ensure the information entering the system is correct, assessment of muscles is crucial before embarking on complex reorganised dentistry.

TMJ

The mechanoreceptors in the TMJ joint appear to play a more significant role in providing information in regard to jaw position and movement (Klineberg 1980).

Soft Tissue Receptors

- *Mucosal and periosteal* – these receptors are more important when teeth are lost, i.e. when wearing a complete denture or an implant-supported prostheses (Jacobs and Van Steenberge 1991).
- *Cutaneous* – the skin contains cutaneous receptors which provide kinaesthetic perceptions, and this has been shown in other parts of the body such as the hand. It is thought that the skin overlying the TMJ may also respond to stretch and therefore provide additional input information regarding condylar movement. There is no direct evidence for this, but we can surmise this during phonetics where the somatosensory input from the facial skin and muscle mechanoreceptors is consistently activated (McClean et al. 1990).

The masticatory system is therefore an all-encompassing, information-gathering and communicative neuromuscular system. The term 'neuromuscular dentistry' was introduced by Dr Bernard Jankelson in 1967 which helps us understand that the masticatory system is a three-dimensional system composed of the TMJ, muscles and teeth with a focus on using transcutaneous electrical nerve stimulators (TENS) to stimulate and relax the muscles, thus providing a physiological rest position and the occlusion was then built around this position. There are many other schools of occlusion and they all recognise that we must assess the TMJ and muscles before rebuilding the teeth because an unhealthy joint does not function in the same way as a healthy one.

So, we are chewing our food happily but when are the teeth touching? Jankelson (1953) stated that 'contact of teeth seldom occurs during the act'. Wassell et al. (2008) state that the time teeth actually touch in total over a 24-hour period is 17.5 minutes.

- 8 minutes empty swallowing contacts – equating to 500 swallowing contacts.
- 9.5 minutes of chewing contacts – the chewing contacts start to occur at the end phase of chewing providing the necessary information that the food is ready to be swallowed – equating to 1800 chewing contacts.

This means that teeth are designed for minimal contact and low forces so when we increase contact time and force, as in parafunction or hypernormal function (nail biting, chewing gum), the teeth can wear, crack or become inflamed (pulpitis), the muscles become inflamed or enlarged, the TMJ becomes inflamed and cartilage can become displaced.

So when do we know when to swallow? When the food is broken down to a size that is small enough for us not to choke and there is variability amongst individuals with regard to size. It was Parmeijer et al. (1970) who showed that the majority of swallowing contacts are in a habitual occlusal position, also called intercuspal position (ICP) or maximum intercuspation (MIP), using intraoral occlusal telemetry devices (a multifrequency transmitter) and less so in centric relation.

Deglutition (Swallowing)

This follows mastication, and is a complex co-ordination of more than 25 pairs of muscles involving the mouth, pharynx, larynx and oesophagus (Miller 1982). The CPG for swallowing is located in the medulla oblongata that contains neurons which trigger, shape, and control the rhythmic swallowing patterns.

Deglutition comprises two phases as discussed by Miller (1982).

1) *Oral preparatory phase* including the pharyngeal phase (voluntary) – the bolus is formed and the positioning of the bolus posteriorly by the extrinsic muscles of the tongue and mylohyoid muscle propels the food further down.
2) *Oesophageal phase* (involuntary) – irreversible once initiated and consists of peristaltic contractions.

Once the food enters the stomach, the process of extracting the nutrients begins. Therefore, the impact of not breaking our food down properly does not just stop at missing teeth and aesthetic concerns; there is a greater impact on the overall health of the patient, especially gut health, and this can lead to disturbed sleep and possible triggers for parafunction.

If the input system is the same (we all have PDMRs, etc.), why is there such variability amongst individuals? The variability starts at the higher order level in the brain within the somatosensory system. This is continuously modulated and is not hardwired but plastic, meaning it has the ability to adapt to functional demand which can be affected by cognitive and emotional factors such as stress, etc. The term 'neuroplasticity' attempts to clarify this and underlines the need to expand our view of occlusion. Just because we have some individuals with greater adaptability, that does not give us carte blanche to perform less than optimal occlusal treatment. Then we have patients who are occlusally hypervigilant whom you would assume have a greater occlusal perception but that doesn't appear to be case; rather, the thoughts and emotions accompanying the altered occlusion appear to be more significant (Klineberg and Eckert 2015).

Phonetics

This is a complex neural network linking an estimated 100 muscles of the respiratory, laryngeal and supraglottal articulatory systems to convert a discretely specified linguistic message to a continuous stream of sounds that can be understood by others (Price 2012). The production of sounds involves the primary motor cortex along several cranial and spinal nerves to the various muscles of respiration and the vocal tract (Jurgens 2002). Most sounds are produced by outgoing air (egressive) and the vocal tracts act as a valve – abduction (opening) provides voiceless sounds and adduction (closing) creates a vibration effect (Martone and Black 1962) which results in voiced sounds. The frequency provides pitch and intensity provides loudness. This is further modified by resonators and articulators. The resonators are the larynx (major) and pharynx (minor) and articulation, which is extremely important in speech sounds, is provided by the lips, tongue and teeth (Elsubeihi et al. 2019). The links with prosthodontics are addressed later in the book.

Cognitive Trap

A dangerous trap that we all have fallen into prevents the dentist from understanding that 'occlusal adjustment' or 'insertion of an occlusal appliance' are not merely 'mechanical' interventions aiming to eliminate premature contacts or to change the occlusion and restore centric relation. Rather, these therapeutic procedures are likely to be accompanied by additional actions that contribute to symptom remission, such as the clinician speaking positively about treatments, providing encouragement and developing trust, reassurance and a supportive relationship (Benedetti and Amanzio 2011).

Conclusion

How do we link all this to what we do on a daily basis?

- Mastication – dynamic contacts – group function, canine guidance.
- Swallowing – static contacts – intercuspal position, maximum intercuspation.

The chapter has focused on the neural pathways involved in occlusion and linked the TMJ, muscles and teeth with the CNS.

References

Benedetti, F. and Amanzio, M. (2011). The placebo response: how words and rituals change the patient's brain. *Patient Educ. Couns.* 84: 413–419.

Byers, M.R. (1985). Sensory innervation of periodontal ligament of rat molar consists of unencapsulated Ruffini-like mechanoreceptors and free nerve endings. *J. Comp. Neurol.* 231: 500–518.

Clark, G.T., Tsukiyama, Y., Baba, K., and Watanabe, T. (1999). Sixty-eight years of experimental occlusal interference studies: what have we learned? *J. Prosthet. Dent.* 82: 704–713.

Elsubeihi, E.S., Elkareimi, Y., and Elbishari, H. (2019). Phonetic considerations in restorative dentistry. *Dent. Update* 46: 880–893.

Herren, P. (1988). Okklusale Taktilität beim bewussten Zusammenbeissen und beim Kauen (Occlusal tactility during conscious biting and during chewing). Thesis, University of Zurich, Zurich.

Jacobs, R. and van Steenberghe, D. (1991). Comparative evaluation of the oral tactile function by means of teeth or implant supported prostheses. *Clin. Oral Implants Res.* 2: 75–80.

Jankelson, B., Hofmann, G.M., and Hendron, J.A. (1953). The physiology of the stomatognathic system. *JADA* 46: 375.

Johnsen, S.E., Svensson, K.G., and Trulsson, M. (2007). Forces applied by anterior and posterior teeth and roles of periodontal afferents during hold-and-split tasks in human subjects. *Exp. Brain Res.* 178 (1): 126–134.

Jurgens, U. (2002). Neural pathways underlying vocal control. *Neurosci. Biobehav. Rev.* 26: 235–258.

Kandel, E.R., Schwartz, J.H., Jessell, T.M. et al. (2012). Principles of Neural Science, 5e, 1709. New York: McGraw-Hill.

Kistemaker, D.A., Van-Soest, A.J.K., Wong, J.D. et al. (2013). Control of position and movement is simplified by combined muscle spindle and Golgi tendon organ feedback. *J. Neurophysiol.* 109: 1126–1139.

Klineberg, I. (1980). Influences of temporomandibular articular mechanoreceptors on functional jaw movements. *J. Oral Rehabil.* 7 (4): 307–317.

Klineberg, I. and Eckert, S. (2015). Functional Occlusion in Restorative Dentistry and Prosthodontics, 1e. St Louis, MO: Mosby.

Lambrichts, I., Creemers, J., and van Steenberghe, D. (1992). Morphology of neural endings in the human periodontal ligament: an electron microscopic study. *J. Periodont. Res.* 27: 191–196.

Lund, J.P. (1991). Mastication and its control by the brain stem. *Crit. Rev. Oral Biol. Med.* 2: 33–64.

Maeda, T., Ochi, K., Nakakura-Ohshima, K. et al. (1999). The Ruffini ending as the primary mechanoreceptor in the periodontal ligament: its morphology, cytochemical features, regeneration, and development. *Crit. Rev. Oral Biol. Med.* 10 (3): 307–327.

Martone, A. and Black, J.M. (1962). An approach to prosthodontics through speech science: part VI. Physiology of speech. *J. Prosthet. Dent.* 12: 409–419.

Matsuo, K. and Palmer, J.B. (2008). Anatomy and physiology of feeding and swallowing: normal and abnormal. *Phys. Med. Rehabil. Clin. North Am.* 19 (4): 691.

McClean, M.D., Dostrovsky, J.O., Lee, L., and Tasker, R.R. (1990). Somatosensory neurons in human thalamus respond to speech-induced orofacial movements. *Brain Res.* 513: 343–347.

12 | *Practical Procedures in Dental Occlusion*

Miller, A.J. (1982). Deglutition. *Physiol. Rev.* 62: 129–184.

Morquette, P., Lavoie, R., Fhima, M.D. et al. (2012). Generation of the masticatory central pattern and its modulation by sensory feedback. *Prog. Neurobiol.* 96 (3): 340–355.

Parmeijer, J.H., Brion, M., Glickman, I., and Roeber, F.W. (1970). Intraoral occlusal telemetry. IV. Tooth contact during swallowing. *J. Prosthet. Dent.* 24 (4): 396–400.

Peyron, M.A., Blanc, O., Lund, J.P., and Woda, A. (2004). Influence of age on adaptability of human mastication. *J. Neurophysiol.* 92: 773–779.

Piancino, M.G., Isola, G., Cannavale, R. et al. (2017). From periodontal mechanoreceptors to chewing motor control: a systematic review. *Arch. Oral Biol.* 78: 109–121.

Plesh, O., Bishop, B., and McCall, W. (1986). Effect of gum hardness on chewing pattern. *Exp. Neurol.* 92: 502.

Price, C.J. (2012). A review and synthesis of the first 20 years of PET and fMRI studies of heard speech, spoken language and reading. *Neuroimage* 62: 816–847.

Randow, K. and Glanz, P.O. (1986). On cantilever loading of vital and non-vital teeth an experimental clinical study. *Acta Odontol. Scand.* 44: 271–277.

Sato, O., Maeda, T., Kobayashi, S. et al. (1988). Innervation of periodontal ligament and dental pulp in the rat incisor: an immunohistochemical investigation of neurofilament protein and glia-specific S-100 protein. *Cell Tissue Res.* 251: 13–21.

Steuer, I. and Guertin, P.A. (2019). Central pattern generators in the brainstem and spinal cord: an overview of basic principles, similarities and differences. *Rev. Neurosci.* 30 (2): 107–164.

Svensson, K.G. and Trulsson, M. (2011). Impaired force control during food holding and biting in subjects with tooth- or implant-supported fixed prostheses. *J. Clin. Periodontol.* 38 (12): 1137–1146.

Svensson, G., Grigoriades, J., and Trulsson, M. (2013). Alterations in intra-oral manipulation and splitting of food by subjects with tooth or implant-supported fixed prostheses. *Clin. Oral Implants Res.* 24: 549–555.

Trulsson, M. and Johansson, R.S. (1996). Forces applied by the incisors and roles of periodontal afferents during food-holding and -biting tasks. *Exp. Brain Res.* 107: 486–496.

Van Lunteren, E. and Dick, T.E. (1997). Muscles of the upper airway and accessory respiratory muscles. In: Neural Control of the Respiratory Muscles (eds. A. Miller, A. Bianchi and B. Bishop), 47–58. Boca Raton, FL: CRC Press.

Wassell, R., Naru, A., Steele, J., and Nohl, F. (2008). Applied Occlusion. New Malden: Quintessence Publishing.

Yabushita, T., Zeredo, J.L., Fujita, K. et al. (2006). Functional adaptability of jaw-muscle spindles after bite-raising. *J. Dent. Res.* 85: 849.

Further Reading

Osterberg, T., Carlsson, G.E., Sundh, V. et al. (2008). Number of teeth – predictor of mortality in 70-year old subjects. *Comm. Dent. Oral Epidemiol.* 36: 258–268.

Trulsson, M. (2007). Force encoding by human periodontal mechanoreceptors during mastication. *Arch. Oral Biol.* 52: 357–360.

3

What's of Use to Me in Practice? Armamentarium, Equipment and Techniques

The Occlusal Examination Tray

Figure 3.1 shows the instruments needed to perform an occlusal examination.

Shimstock Foil

Function, Features, and Practical Tips

This is a metal foil for occlusal testing (thickness = 8 µm) (Figure 3.2). It is used as a feeler gauge between occluding teeth to check firmness of occlusal contacts in comparison with those on the selected index teeth. When you fit a crown, both restoration and adjacent teeth should hold the shimstock firmly in intercuspal position (ICP).

Shimstock can also be used to ensure the accuracy of the mounting of the models. This can be checked with shimstock such that the intraoral contacts and those on the casts coincide (Figure 3.3).

- Anterior teeth often have light shimstock contacts which should be kept light after restoration.
- Shimstock contacts that are obviously firmer than the adjacent teeth usually indicate heavy occlusal loading.

Articulating Papers

Function, Features, and Practical Tips

- Carbon paper used to mark occlusal contacts on a surface of teeth, restoration or prosthesis (Figure 3.4).

Practical Procedures in Dental Occlusion, First Edition. Ziad Al-Ani and Riaz Yar.
© 2022 John Wiley & Sons Ltd. Published 2022 by John Wiley & Sons Ltd.
Companion website: www.wiley.com/go/al-ani-and-riaz/dental-occlusion

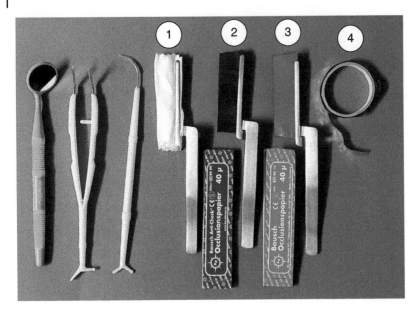

Figure 3.1 The occlusal examination tray. (1) Paper tissues held in Miller's forceps for drying occlusal surfaces of teeth before marking them, (2) 40 μ blue articulating paper held in Miller's forceps, (3) 40 μ red articulating paper held in Miller's forceps, and (4) Shimstock foil.

(a)   (b)

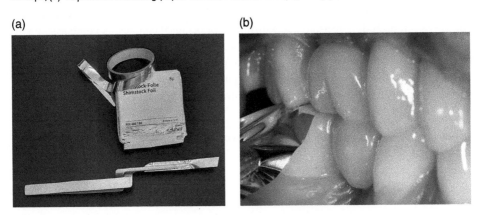

Figure 3.2 (a) Shimstock foil and (b) Shimstock in use as a feeler gauge between occluding teeth.

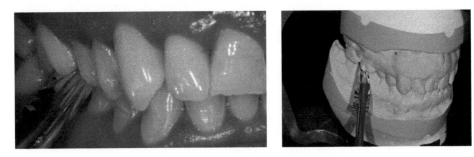

Figure 3.3 Shimstock can be used to ensure the accuracy of the mounting of the models.

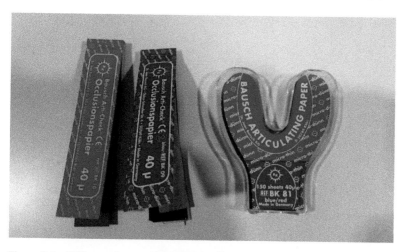

Figure 3.4 Different shapes of articulating papers.

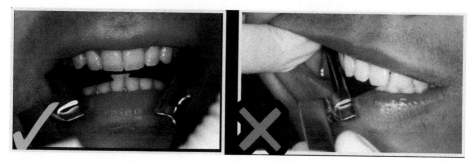

Figure 3.5 The articulating papers must be placed simultaneously on the two sides.

- Use thin articulating papers as they minimise contact artefacts and clearly indicate tooth contact details by marking only the small points of true contact. Thick paper will mark a large area surrounding the point of contact. Articulating paper which overmarks teeth makes interpretation difficult (see Chapter 4).
- Use different coloured tapes for identifying specific tooth contacts and to allow comparisons to be made.
- Teeth should be dried to allow articulating papers to mark the teeth.
- Some articulating papers contain an emulsifier which facilitates the process of marking shiny occlusal surfaces such as metal and ceramic restorations.
- The articulating papers must be placed simultaneously on the two sides. Placement on only one side will result in displacement of the mandible toward the side where the occlusal paper is placed (Figure 3.5). Two Millers forceps should be used to hold two articulating papers both sides when marking contacts in ICP. Alternatively, a Y-type articulating paper holder (Figure 3.6) can be used to hold one wide square-shaped or horseshoe articulating paper which can be applied simultaneously on both sides.

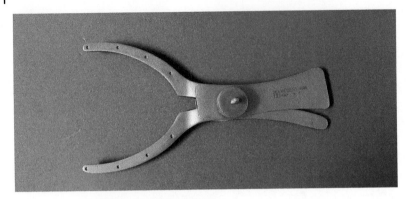

Figure 3.6   Y-type articulating paper holder.

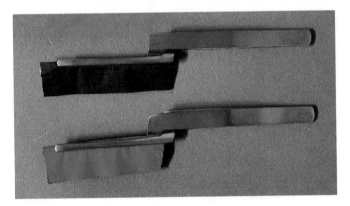

Figure 3.7   Articulating papers held by Miller's forceps.

Miller's Forceps

Function, Features, and Practical Tips

- Miller's forceps securely grip the entire length of the articulating paper while checking the occlusion (Figure 3.7). They stop the paper crumpling.
- When checking occlusion on posterior teeth, the articulating paper should be about 5 mm longer than the forceps to avoid discomfort caused by the patient closing down on the end of the forceps.

Registration Media and Techniques

The patient's occlusion should be recorded before any treatment is started. The construction of an indirect restoration requires the transfer of anatomical information from the clinician to the dental laboratory technician. This requires accurate models of the patient's teeth and an occlusal registration, centric jaw relation and facebow record.

Occlusal registration is a physical record which, by determining the jaw relationships (existing or desired), allows for transfer of the upper and lower models to the articulator in that jaw relationship.

The loss of interocclusal contact created by preparation of a tooth for a single unit restoration is unlikely to detract from the ease with which working and opposing casts can be located in ICP.

It is worth taking the opportunity of examining the ease with which any study casts can be located by hand before deciding whether an occlusal registration is needed. Often (perhaps even usually) you are better with nothing at all. 'The best occlusal registration is no registration.'

It is recognised that all materials and techniques for producing occlusal registration have some level of inaccuracy. The occlusal registration must allow accurate articulation of the casts and the properties of the registration must allow complete dimensional stability.

Placing a layer of wax between the casts to help to locate them can often result in them failing to seat into ICP (inaccuracies) and the 'squash bite' technique using pink sheet wax is not recommended because it readily fails under pressure and has insufficient strength to maintain accuracy (Figure 3.8).

Polyvinyl Siloxane Syringable Materials

A very detailed silicone occlusal record including embrasures and gingival tissues can prevent it seating properly on the cast and the combination of a very detailed silicone occlusal registration and less detailed stone cast, particularly of the occlusal fissures, has meant that

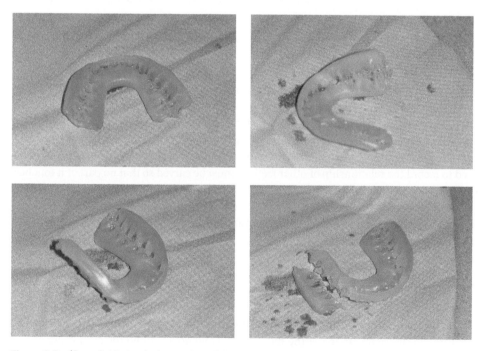

Figure 3.8 'Squash bite' technique using pink sheet wax is not recommended.

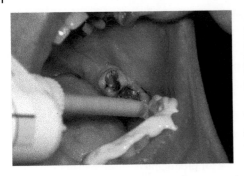
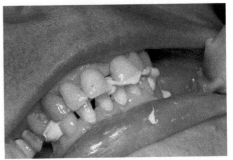

Figure 3.9 Full arch detailed occlusal registration.

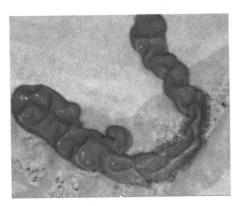
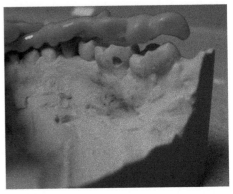

Figure 3.10 Excessive details on the occlusal registration may hinder seating on a stone cast.

the record will not seat (Figure 3.9). Moreover, the excessive detail may well hinder seating on a stone cast (Figure 3.10).

If possible, the bite registration material should only be used between the prepared tooth and its antagonists, not to take a full arch occlusal registration. Record the tips of cusps or preparations, avoiding capturing fissure patterns and any soft tissue contact as much as possible. A carefully trimmed registration leaving only areas essential for location and restricted to the area of tooth preparation is favourable. If a bite registration is going to be used to record the relationship of other teeth, it must be carved so that no part of it touches the models of the mucosal surfaces (Figure 3.11).

Digital technology can now be utilised for the process of obtaining interocclusal recording and with the introduction of new intraoral scanner systems, virtual bite registrations can be accurately obtained (Figure 3.12).

Centric Relation Record

A centric relation (CR) registration is taken by inducing relaxation of the masticatory muscles through the gentle arcing of the mandible up and down, along the closing arc of the terminal hinge axis, using gentle bimanual manipulation while the patient is supine. It has

(a)

(b)

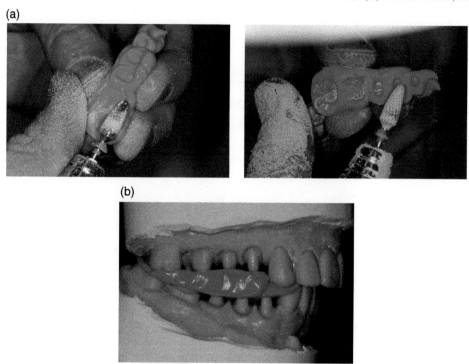

Figure 3.11   A carefully trimmed registration limited to the area of tooth preparation is preferable.

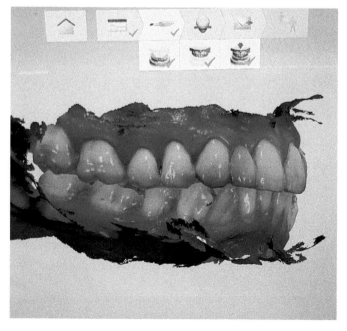

Figure 3.12   Virtual bite registrations can be accurately obtained using intraoral scanner systems.
Source: Al-Ani Z, Gray RJM. (2021). Temporomandibular Disorders: A Problem-Based Approach, 2nd edn. John Wiley & Sons Ltd, Chichester.

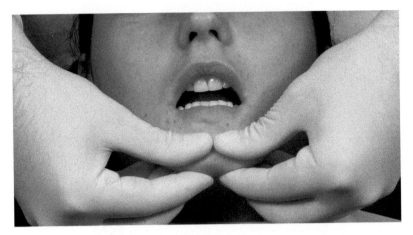

Figure 3.13 Passive manipulation of the mandible of a supine patient used for achieving centric relation. *Source:* Al-Ani Z, Gray RJM. (2021). Temporomandibular Disorders: A Problem-Based Approach, 2nd edn. John Wiley & Sons Ltd, Chichester.

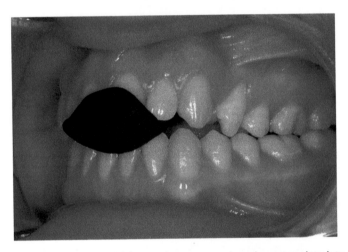

Figure 3.14 Greenstick impression compound used as a template into which the patient is able to close in centric relation after manipulation of the mandible to centric relation. *Source:* Al-Ani Z, Gray RJM. (2021). Temporomandibular Disorders: A Problem-Based Approach, 2nd edn. John Wiley & Sons Ltd, Chichester.

been suggested that the patient's mandible describes a perfect arc during manipulation, which gives the operator the confidence that the terminal hinge axis of the mandible has been found (Figure 3.13).

A small quantity of warm, soft, greenstick impression compound is placed over the palatal and incisal surfaces of the upper anterior teeth during this manipulation, until the lower anterior teeth make indentations in the material. This is used as a template when it has cooled and hardened to assist the patient in reproducibly closing into centric relation (Figure 3.14).

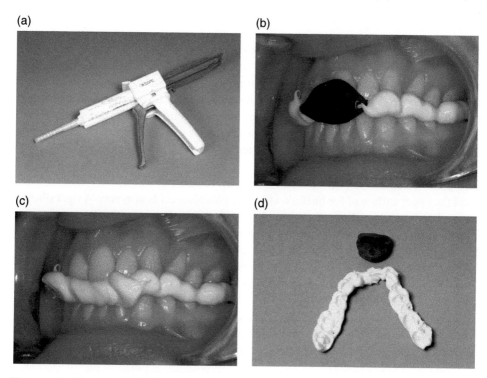

Figure 3.15 (a–d) A suitable bite registration material is syringed between the posterior teeth, with the greenstick impression compound used as a template for achieving a complete centric relation. *Source:* Al-Ani Z, Gray RJM. (2021). Temporomandibular Disorders: A Problem-Based Approach, 2nd edn. John Wiley & Sons Ltd, Chichester.

A suitable bite registration material (polyvinyl siloxane, PVS) is then syringed into the interocclusal posterior gap bilaterally. Once this has hardened, the greenstick is subsequently replaced by a further mix of bite registration material on the anterior teeth, using the set material on the posterior teeth as a template to obtain a full, single, horseshoe centric relation registration (Figure 3.15a–d). This centric relation registration with the impressions and facebow transfer jig record is sent to the laboratory, and the models of the arches are mounted in the semi-adjustable articulator.

Facebow Registration

Function, Features, and Practical Tips

This relates the upper model of the dental arch to the hinges of the articulator in the same spatial relationship as exists between the maxillary teeth and the temporomandibular joints (TMJs). This also helps to determine that, during construction of the splint, any opening or closing of the semi-adjustable articulator occurs along the same arc as in the mouth.

Using the Facebow: Step by Step

Locating and Marking a Reference Point on the Patient's Face

Figure 3.16 shows Earbow and accessories needed for facebow registration. An anterior reference point, along with the other two posterior points, needs to be established first for an accurate facebow record. The position of the anterior reference point is measured 43 mm from the incisal edge of the central or lateral incisor, toward the inner corner of the eye. The notched-out area of the 'reference plane locator' is used to make this measurement. Mark the anterior reference point on the patient's face using a marker (Figure 3.17).

Taking the Facebow Registration (Assembling the Earbow on the Patient)

Load the upper surface of the bitefork with two thicknesses of beauty wax. A rigid silicone bite registration material may also be used as bitefork recording material (Figure 3.18).

Soften the wax to a very soft consistency in warm water or over an open flame. With the bitefork arm projecting to the patient's right, place it on to the patient's upper teeth, aligning midline to obtain a light indexing impression of the maxillary teeth. Stabilise this by instructing the patient to hold it steady using the thumbs. Let the material harden before proceeding (Figures 3.19 and 3.20).

Loosen the centre wheel on the earbow and the finger screws on the transfer jig. Slide the transfer jig onto the bitefork arm and guide the earbow into the patient's ears with their help. Pull the earbow together and tighten the centre wheel, ensuring even placement in both ear canals (Figure 3.21).

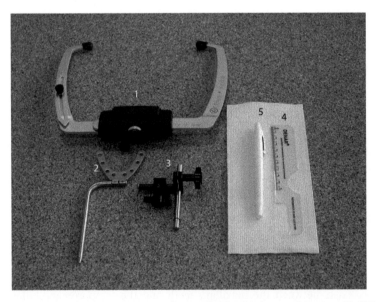

Figure 3.16　Earbow and accessories needed for facebow registration. (1) Slidematic U-shape earbow, (2) dentate bitefork, (3) transfer jig, (4) reference plane locator, and (5) marker pen. *Source:* Al-Ani Z, Gray RJM. (2021). Temporomandibular Disorders: A Problem-Based Approach, 2nd edn. John Wiley & Sons Ltd, Chichester.

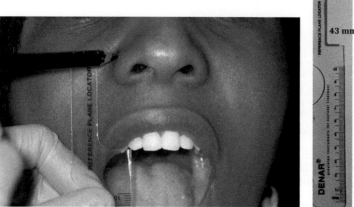

Figure 3.17 Marking the anterior reference point. *Source:* Photo 3.17a is taken from Al-Ani Z, Gray RJM. (2021). Temporomandibular Disorders: A Problem-Based Approach, 2nd edn. John Wiley & Sons Ltd, Chichester.

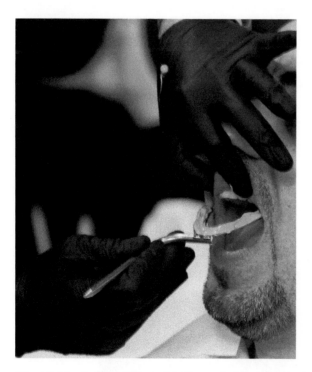

Figure 3.18 A silicone bite registration material can be used as a bitefork recording medium.

Raise or lower the bow so that the pointer aligns with the anterior reference point on the patient's face. You can also look through a slot in the bow to verify this. Engage the transfer jig in the earbow and tighten finger screws 1 and 2 on the transfer jig, being careful not to torque the earbow.

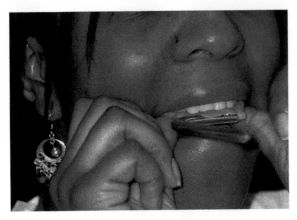

Figure 3.19   The bitefork is placed on to the patient's upper teeth and stabilised by the patient's thumbs. *Source:* Al-Ani Z, Gray RJM. (2021). Temporomandibular Disorders: A Problem-Based Approach, 2nd edn. John Wiley & Sons Ltd, Chichester.

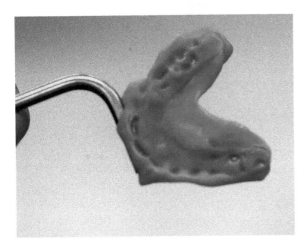

Figure 3.20   Light indexing impression of the maxillary teeth on the bitefork. *Source:* Al-Ani Z, Gray RJM. (2021). Temporomandibular Disorders: A Problem-Based Approach, 2nd edn. John Wiley & Sons Ltd, Chichester.

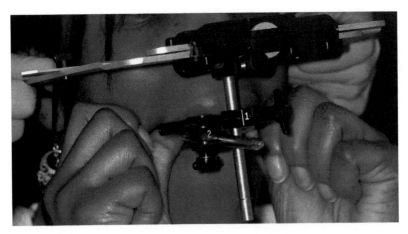

Figure 3.21   The earbow is guided into the patient's ears. *Source:* Al-Ani Z, Gray RJM. (2021). Temporomandibular Disorders: A Problem-Based Approach, 2nd edn. John Wiley & Sons Ltd, Chichester.

Always ensure that the numbers '1' and '2' are the correct way up and facing you (Figure 3.22).

Have the patient stand and, looking at the patient from the front, verify that the bow is horizontal to the horizon and the patient's pupils. Some facebow systems include a bubble level which will help with this (Figure 3.23). Adjust as necessary and retighten finger screws 1 and 2 as necessary (Figure 3.24).

Loosen the centre screw on the earbow, slide open and remove the entire earbow assembly, transfer jig and bitefork from the patient (Figure 3.25). Detach the earbow from the transfer jig assembly. Carefully tighten finger screws 1 and 2, making sure not to torque or

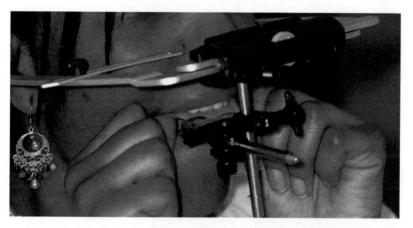

Figure 3.22   The pointer is aligned with the anterior reference point on the patient's face. *Source:* Al-Ani Z, Gray RJM. (2021). Temporomandibular Disorders: A Problem-Based Approach, 2nd edn. John Wiley & Sons Ltd, Chichester.

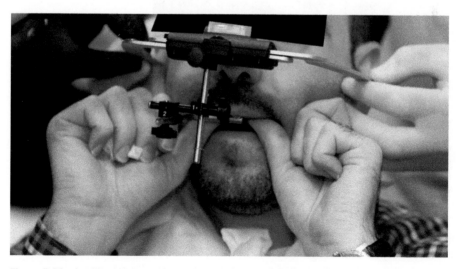

Figure 3.23   Looking at the patient from the front, verify that the bow is horizontal to the horizon and the patient's pupils. A bubble level can help in this verification.

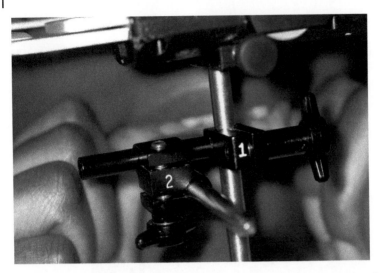

Figure 3.24 Finger screws 1 and 2 are securely tightened before removing the earbow. *Source:* Al-Ani Z, Gray RJM. (2021). Temporomandibular Disorders: A Problem-Based Approach, 2nd edn. John Wiley & Sons Ltd, Chichester.

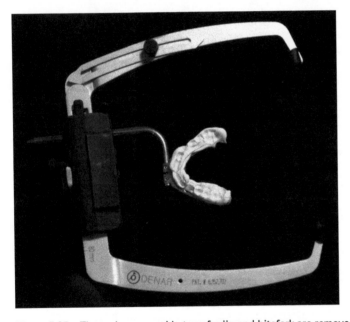

Figure 3.25 The earbow assembly, transfer jig and bitefork are removed from the patient.

change the transfer jig assembly (Figure 3.26). Disinfect the transfer jig assembly and send it to the laboratory for mounting.

The transfer jig and the fork are then assembled on the semi-adjustable articulator using a mounting shoe which replaces the incisal table of the articulator (Figure 3.27).

(a)

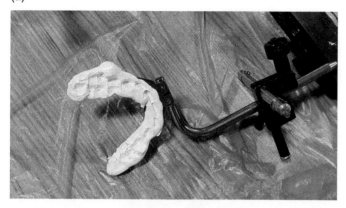

(b)

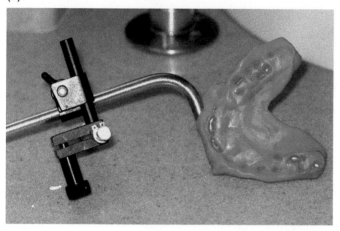

Figure 3.26 (a) Transfer jig after detachment from the earbow, (b) screws 1 and 2 should be tightened before transferring to the laboratory. *Source:* Photo 3.26b is taken from Al-Ani Z, Gray RJM. (2021). Temporomandibular Disorders: A Problem-Based Approach, 2nd edn. John Wiley & Sons Ltd, Chichester.

Articulators

Function, Features, and Practical Tips

Simple Hinge Articulators (Non-anatomical Occlude), Semi-Adjustable, and Average-Value Articulators

Simple hinge articulators (non-anatomic occlude) (Figure 3.28) provide a single hinge movement without lateral movements and are unable to accept facebow transfer. They therefore have a limited application and are only suitable for individual crowns in a Class I incisor relationship as the ICP recordings are an approximation. When more than one tooth is involved in the restorations or when these teeth are involved in the anterior guidance, these types of articulators will produce inaccurate occlusion.

(a)

(b)

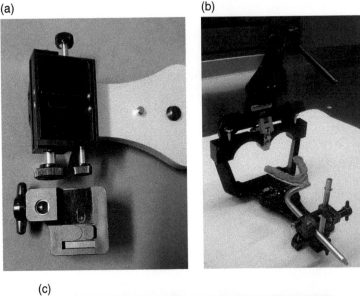

(c)

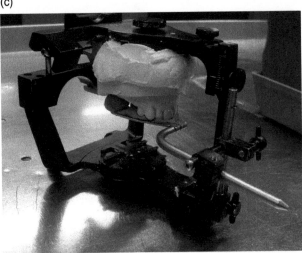

Figure 3.27 (a) A mounting shoe replaces the incisal guide table. (b) Transfer jig and fork are assembled on a semi-adjustable articulator using a mounting shoe. (c) Upper cast attached to upper member of the articulator with mounting stone.

The arc of opening on the simple hinge articulator is different from that of a patient as the hinge is closer to the teeth on the model than the TMJ would be to the teeth in the mouth and the distance of the upper arch to the intercondylar axis is much less than in the patient. In a patient, the radius from transverse horizontal axis to tooth tip is in the region of 65 mm. In the non-anatomical articulator, however, this distance is about 40 mm. In anatomical articulators such as semi-adjustable articulators, this distance is relatively close to the measures in the patient (Figure 3.29).

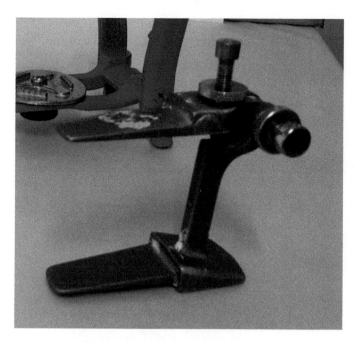

Figure 3.28   Simple hinge articulators (non-anatomical occlude).

When using a non-anatomical articulator for constructing indirect restorations, some adjustment of the cuspal inclines of restorations is usually needed on closure to compensate for the inaccuracy of the articulator. The adjusted restorations will tend to have cusps with reduced height and shallow angles, giving them a relatively flat appearance (Figure 3.30). If there is a deep bite with heavy anterior teeth contacts, as, for instance, in an Angles class II division II case, then the anterior restorations would be very difficult without the use of facebow and semi-adjustable articulator. Similarly, posterior restorations would be very difficult without the use of facebow and semi-adjustable articulator in cases of absence of incisor contacts as in an Angles class III or anterior open bite when posterior teeth form the guiding surfaces.

In contrast, semi-adjustable articulators allow adjustment to simulate mandibular movements (Figure 3.31). They accept facebow transfer, ensuring that the arc of opening and closing of the mandible is replicated in the articulator as well as giving an indication of the position of the occlusal plane. They can reproduce jaw movements. These articulators, therefore, are recommended for most dental restorations.

Arcon type semi-adjustable articulators have their condyles in the anatomically correct position on the lower member, simplifying the TMJs. These types of articulators are preferred for construction of indirect restorations with accurate occlusion (Figure 3.32).

Parts and Components of Semi-Adjustable Articulator

Figure 3.33 illustrates the parts and components of the Denar® (Mk II) semi-adjustable articulator.

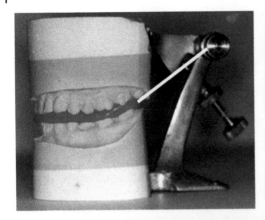
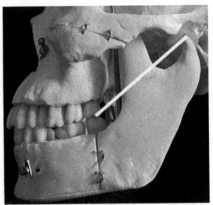
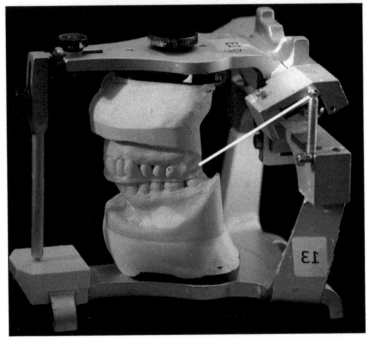

Figure 3.29 Comparison of the radius from transverse horizontal axis to tooth tip between the skull, a non-anatomical articulator and a semi-adjustable articulator.

The intercondylar distance in semi-adjustable articulators is usually fixed at a width of 110 mm representing the average intercondylar distance. Some articulators use different intercondylar width settings (Figure 3.34).

Condylar inclination (condylar guidance) is the angle made by the movement of the condyle down and forward onto the articular eminence (Figure 3.35). On a semi-adjustable articulator, this is usually set at 25–30° (Figure 3.36). This will enable the technician to produce restorations with low cusps and easy to disclude in excursions. In some cases when more posterior teeth separation is needed, this setting of the condylar guidance can be increased (Figure 3.37).

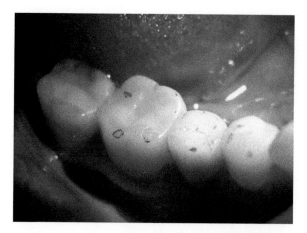

Figure 3.30 Restorations constructed on a non-anatomical articulator. Note the considerable adjustments of the heights of the cusps to compensate for the inaccuracy of the articulator.

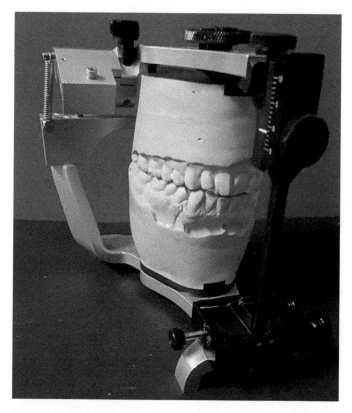

Figure 3.31 Semi-adjustable articulators allow adjustment to simulate mandibular movements.

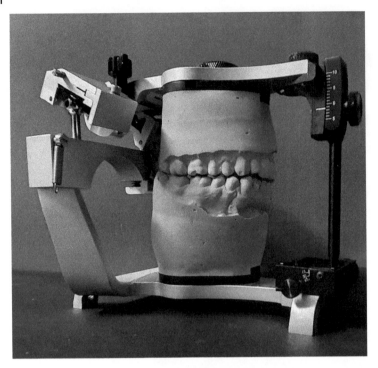

Figure 3.32   Arcon type semi-adjustable articulators have their condyles in the anatomically correct position on the lower member, simplifying the TMJs.

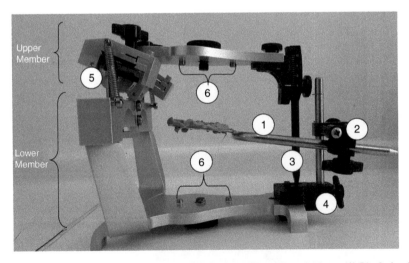

Figure 3.33   Parts and components of the semi-adjustable articulator. (1) Bitefork with silicone registration material, (2) transfer jig, (3) incisal pin, (4) mounting shoe, (5) articulator condyle (Arcon type), and (6) screw and lugs used to attach the baseplates for mounting the casts.

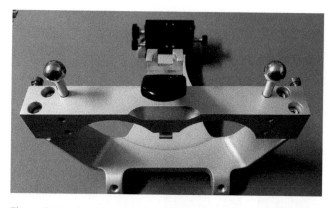

Figure 3.34 The intercondylar distance in semi-adjustable articulators is usually fixed at a width of 110 mm.

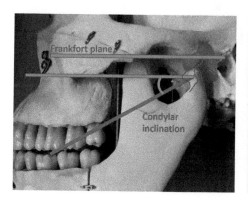
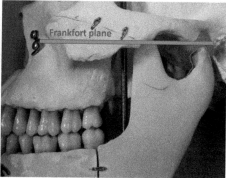

Figure 3.35 Condylar inclination (condylar guidance) is the angle made by the movement of the condyle down and forward onto the articular eminence.

In the lateral excursions, the head of the condyle on the non-working side (NWS) moves forward, downwards and medially. The angle which is produced by this progressive movement is known as the 'Bennett angle' (Figure 3.38). In most semi-adjustable articulators, the Bennett angle is usually set at a value of 15°. In some articulator systems, this value is adjusted midway between 5° and 10° (Figure 3.39).

The movement of the condyle on the working side (WS) is called 'immediate side shift' or 'Bennett movement' and is usually set at 0 (Figure 3.40).

In the lateral excursions on the semi-adjustable articulator, the rotating condyle (on the WS) moves outwards along the distal wall of the fossa element. The orbiting condyle (on the NWS), however, moves inwards and forwards (guided by the medial wall of the fossa element) (Figure 3.41).

Average-value articulators are less accurate than semi-adjustable articulators with values fixed for the intercondylar distance (110 mm), condylar guidance (25°) and Bennett angle (7°) and no immediate side shift. These types of articulators are ideal for fabricating single crowns and minimal unit restorations.

(a)

(b)

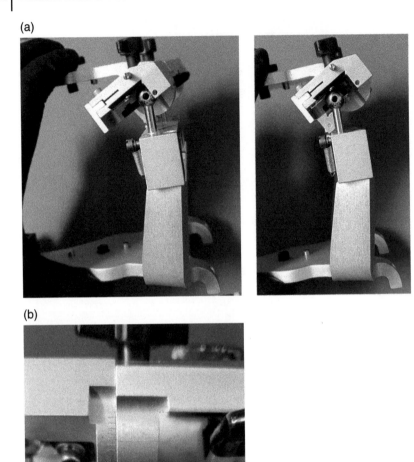

Figure 3.36   (a) Condylar guidance on a semi-adjustable articulator. The condylar ball runs down the superior wall in protrusive movement. (b) Condylar guidance is usually set at 25° on a semi-adjustable articulator.

Fully adjustable articulators are very sophisticated devices which allow closer reproduction of condylar movements but are rarely used. They need a pantographic facebow to record the terminal hinge axis and the position and movement of the condyles. Condylar inserts can be used to duplicate the curved anatomy of the glenoid fossa (Figure 3.42).

Condylar guidance = 25°

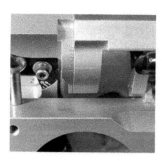

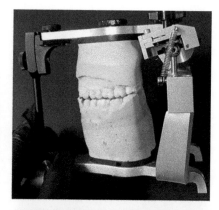

Disclusion of posterior teeth in protrusion

Condylar guidance = 50°

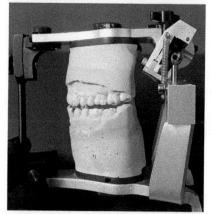

More Disclusion of posterior teeth in protrusion

Condylar guidance = 5°

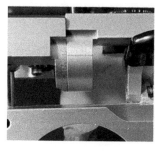

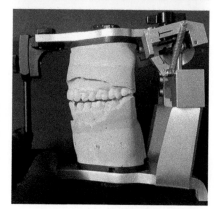

Disclusion disappears and posterior teeth in contact

Figure 3.37 The effect of altering the condylar guidance on the posterior teeth disclusion.

How to Make a Stabilisation Splint (SS)

This full-coverage hard acrylic splint (Figure 3.43) provides a removable ideal occlusion which means in static occlusion, centric occlusion occurs in centric relation and in dynamic occlusion, anterior guidance at the front of the mouth free from posterior interferences.

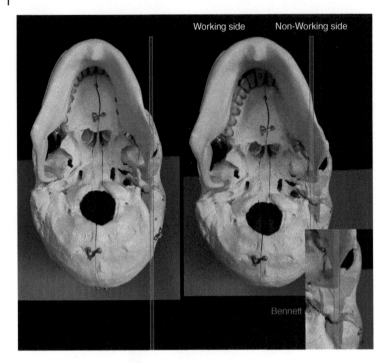

Figure 3.38   Bennett angle.

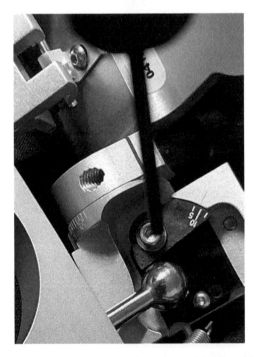

Figure 3.39   Bennett angle set in a semi-adjustable articulator.

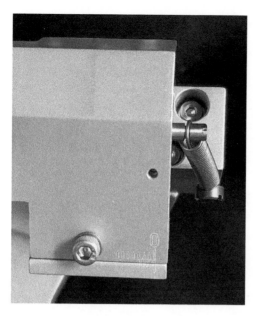

Figure 3.40   Bennett movement set in a semi-adjustable articulator.

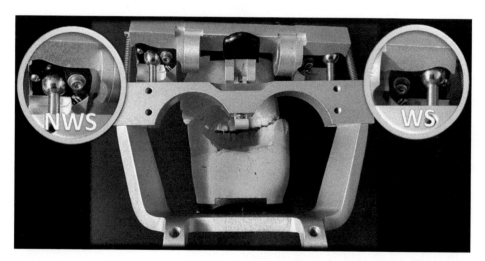

Figure 3.41   Movements of working side and non-working side condyles in a semi-adjustable articulator.

The use of this splint may be considered in various clinical conditions such as management of temporomandibular joint disorders, diagnosis of occlusal disease, stabilisation of the occlusal scheme prior to advanced restorative care provision, including the assessment of patient tolerance to an occlusal scheme, with an altered occlusal vertical dimension. In addition, this splint can be considered as a valuable management option in cases of pathological tooth wear as well as in the management of parafunctional (bruxist) activity.

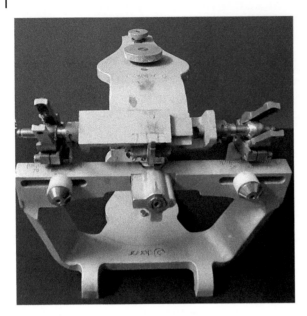

Figure 3.42   Fully adjustable articulator.

(a)   (b)

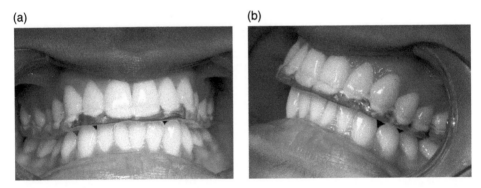

Figure 3.43   Stabilisation splint (Michigan splint).

Practical Steps of Making an SS

The first step is to obtain upper and lower models of the patient's dental arches which are cast from alginate impressions using Die-stone.

Facebow Registration

This relates the upper model of the dental arch to the hinges of the articulator in the same spatial relationship as exists between the maxillary teeth and the TMJs. This helps to determine that, during construction of the splint, any opening or closing of the semi-adjustable articulator occurs along the same arc as in the mouth (see Section 'Facebow Registration').

Centric Relation Registration and Mounting the Casts in CR

Please refer to Section 'Centric Relation Record' on how to make centric relation registration and for the practical procedures of mounting the casts on a semi-adjustable articulator using this registration.

Mounting the Casts on a Semi-adjustable Articulator

The casts are now mounted on a semi-adjustable articulator and a SS is constructed in centric relation jaw position (Figure 3.44). Adequate relief of undercuts and initial polishing are carried out in the laboratory to ensure easy seating of the splint (Figure 3.45).

Fitting a Stabilisation Splint

It will take approximately an hour to fit and balance the splint in the patient's mouth. The splint will be delivered from the laboratory with adequate relief of undercuts to ensure easy seating. The stabilisation splint should be relined with autopolymerising acrylic, intraorally at the chairside, to provide good and positive retention (Figure 3.46).

During relining, the acrylic is applied to the fitting surface of the splint which is then placed on to the teeth and fully seated. The splint must be removed from the mouth before

(a) (b) (c)

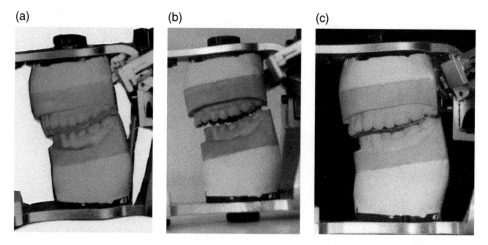

Figure 3.44 Upper and lower models are mounted on a semi-adjustable articulator and a stabilisation splint is constructed in centric relation jaw position, here on the lower model. (a) The models with the bite registration, (b) the models with this registration removed, and (c) the models with the splint inserted. *Source:* Al-Ani Z, Gray RJM. (2021). Temporomandibular Disorders: A Problem-Based Approach, 2nd edn. John Wiley & Sons Ltd, Chichester.

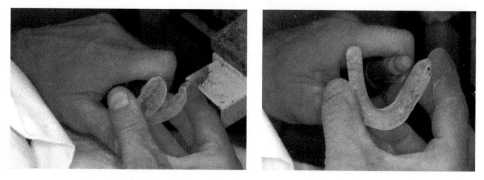

Figure 3.45 Adequate relief of undercuts and initial polishing are carried out in the laboratory. *Source:* Al-Ani Z, Gray RJM. (2021). Temporomandibular Disorders: A Problem-Based Approach, 2nd edn. John Wiley & Sons Ltd, Chichester.

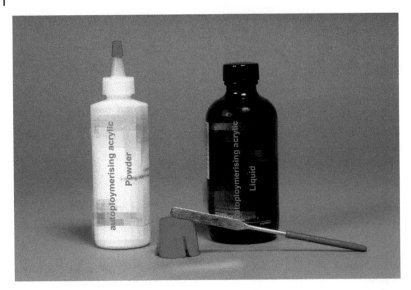

Figure 3.46   Autopolymerising acrylic is used to reline a stabilisation splint intraorally at the chairside to provide positive retention. *Source:* Al-Ani Z, Gray RJM. (2021). Temporomandibular Disorders: A Problem-Based Approach, 2nd edn. John Wiley & Sons Ltd, Chichester.

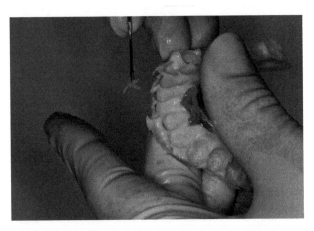

Figure 3.47   The SS was relined with autoploymerising acrylic intraorally at the chairside to provide good and positive retention. The splint must be removed from the mouth before the acrylic has fully set and, when it has set, any excess is removed. *Source:* Al-Ani Z, Gray RJM. (2021). Temporomandibular Disorders: A Problem-Based Approach, 2nd edn. John Wiley & Sons Ltd, Chichester.

the acrylic has fully set and when it has set, any excess is removed using an acrylic trimmer in a straight handpiece. It should then be tried to ensure that it is not too tight but has good retention (Figure 3.47).

Central relation occlusion (CRO) is then established by adjusting the splint, after marking the occlusal contacts using articulating paper until a balanced series of posterior centric stops has been produced. During this procedure, the splint is inserted into the mouth, and

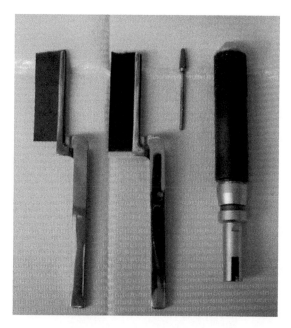

Figure 3.48 Thin articulating papers (two different colours) and straight handpiece with grinding stones are used for adjusting the stabilisation splint.

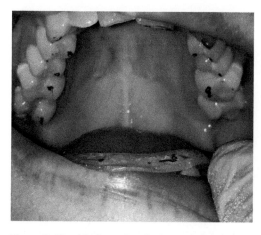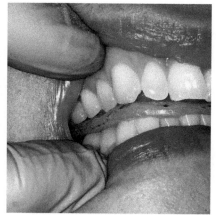

Figure 3.49 A balanced occlusion should be provided between the splint and one cusp tip of every opposing tooth, distally from the canines.

the patient's mandible is gently tapped up and down with the articulating paper interposed between the surface of the splint and the opposing teeth. The splint is then removed and any necessary adjustments are made (Figure 3.48).

Balancing commences by ensuring that the opposing canines touch in centric relation. A balanced occlusion should be provided between the splint and one cusp tip of every opposing tooth, distally from the canines (Figure 3.49).

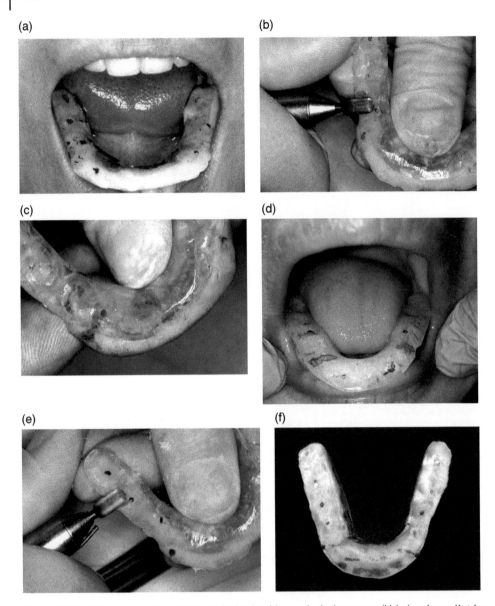

Figure 3.50 (a) Centric relation stops marked using blue articulating paper, (b) balancing splint by adjusting contacts, (c) development of canine guidance using red articulating paper, (d) canine guidance (red), (e) posterior interferences marked and removed, and (f) balanced splint. *Source:* Al-Ani Z, Gray RJM. (2021). Temporomandibular Disorders: A Problem-Based Approach, 2nd edn. John Wiley & Sons Ltd, Chichester.

Repetitive adjustments of the splint are made after marking the occlusal contacts with thin articulating paper, until a full range of centric stops has been achieved.

Ideal anterior guidance (against the opposing canines and incisors) is developed during lateral excursions, and all posterior interferences, on both the working and non-working sides, are marked and removed.

The easy way to ensure that there are no posterior interferences is to have a steep ramp anteriorly, against which the canines slide. This is unnecessary and undesirable, however, as patients find it easier to move laterally on shallow anterior guidance with minimal separation of the posterior teeth.

Once the crossover canine position has been reached, when the lower canine in lateral mandibular excursion has moved lateral to the maxillary canine, the splint is adjusted so that the anterior guidance is transferred to the central incisors, which provide most of the guidance during protrusive movements. As a consequence of wearing the splint, and with the passage of time, muscle relaxation may allow the mandible to adopt a new position. The splint will then need further rebalancing to this new position, until eventually a reproducible centric relation position is established (Figure 3.50).

Further Reading

Al-Ani, Z. and Gray, R.J.M. (2021). Temporomandibular Disorders: A Problem-Based Approach, 2nd edn. Chichester: John Wiley & Sons Ltd.

Davies, S. and Gray, R. (2002). *A Clinical Guide to Occlusion*. London: British Dental Association.

Galeković, N.H., Fugošić, V., Braut, V., and Ćelić, R. (2017). Reproducibility of centric relation techniques by means of condyle position analysis. *Acta Stomatol. Croat.* 51: 13–21.

Keshvad, A. and Winstanley, R.B. (2003). Comparison of the replicability of routinely used centric relation registration techniques. *J. Prosthodont.* 12: 90–101.

Moufti, M.A., Lilico, J.T., and Wassell, R.W. (2007). How to make a well fitting stabilization splint. *Dent. Update* 34: 398–408.

Nohl, F., Steele, J., and Wassell, R. (2002). Crowns and other extra-coronal restorations: aesthetic control. *Br. Dent. J.* 192: 443–450.

Wassell, R., Naru, A., Steele, J., and Nohl, F. (2015). *Applied Occlusion*, 2e. London: Quintessence.

Wilson, P.H. and Banerjee, A. (2004). Recording the retruded contact position: a review of clinical techniques. *Br. Dent. J.* 196: 395–402. quiz 426.

4

I Don't Know What I Am Recording. Where Are the True Contacts?

Scenario

The patient has lost an upper right premolar crown and requires a restoration.

Rationale

Occlusion in simple terms means the contacts between teeth in both a static and dynamic relationship but it is also one part of the masticatory system (Figure 4.1).

The process of assessing occlusion uses the acronym STOP. A preassessment of the occlusion is crucial to ensure we conform safely whether in centric occlusion or centric relation. This process utilises our senses to reduce errors because each element has limitations.

S – Survey – visual assessment using coloured paper to analyse contacts.
T – Touch – fremitus.
O – Observe and listen – sounds of the teeth touching before and after.
P – Patient feedback.

The key to understanding occlusion is occlusal morphology – where the teeth meet in different skeletal molar, canine relationship = occlusal contacts.

Applying this key is next.

- Occlusal contacts – in static and dynamic.
- Preassessment – using correct equipment.
- How to adjust – if not correct.

Occlusal Morphology

The terminology of morphology is a starting point to aid understanding of occlusion (Figure 4.2). There are typically two types of occlusal contact arrangements (variabilities exist where this is an arch discrepancy causing crossbites or overcrowding).

- Cusp tip – fossa = tooth – tooth contact
- Cusp tip – marginal ridge = tooth – two teeth contact

Practical Procedures in Dental Occlusion, First Edition. Ziad Al-Ani and Riaz Yar.
© 2022 John Wiley & Sons Ltd. Published 2022 by John Wiley & Sons Ltd.
Companion website: www.wiley.com/go/al-ani-and-riaz/dental-occlusion

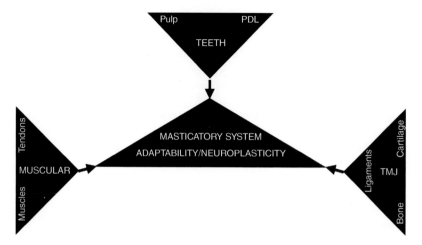

Figure 4.1 The masticatory system and its components.

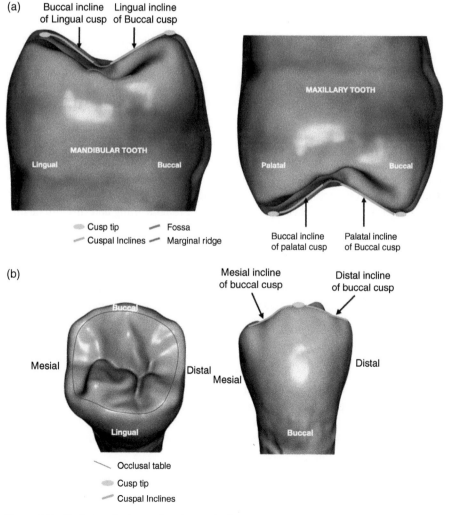

Figure 4.2 Basic terminology related to occlusion.

This reinforces the point that teeth function as a minimum in pairs so when we lose a tooth through extraction, we lose a functioning pair and when we replace a missing tooth, we increase a functional pair. This point aids communication with patients when discussing the loss or replacement of a tooth.

The cuspal anatomy is broken down further as follows.

- Upper arch – palatal cusps are called *supporting* (other terms used in the literature are working or functional).
- Buccal cusps are called *non-supporting* (other terms are non-working or non-functional but strictly this is untrue – all cusps are functional in mastication).
- Lower arch – buccal cusps are called *supporting*. Lingual cusps are called *non-supporting*.

What do we mean by supporting, working and functional?

- These cusps are involved in providing functional contacts when masticating and therefore aid the breakdown of food.
- They maintain occlusal stability, thus supporting the mandible and the occlusal vertical dimension (OVD).
- They provide guidance for the mandible during mastication to come into centric occlusion (maximum intercuspal position).

Does that mean that the non-supporting, working or functional cusps have no role? The terminology suggests this but the buccal and lingual cusps are equally essential.

- They aid mastication by providing a space to contain the food and allow for efficient breakdown (Figure 4.3).
- They provide guidance for the mandible during mastication to come into centric occlusion (maximum intercuspal position).
- They protect the soft tissues – in the upper arch the buccal mucosa and in the lower arch the tongue; hence patients will complain of cheek or tongue biting and this will be due to incorrect cuspal anatomy.

What is the minimum number of occlusal contacts required for stability of the dentition? The evidence is minimal and the variation is high. The textbooks have provided complicated systems to provide occlusal contacts such as the tripodisation theory which suggests that there must be a three-point contact between a cusp and fossa. This is difficult to achieve but more importantly, it is not stable and will be lost with tooth wear, tooth movement and remodelling within the temporomandibular joint (TMJ), etc.

Wiskott and Belser (1995) suggest that no natural dentition presents occlusal contacts as described in many texts so with this point in mind, we are providing a guide which is simple to achieve and will provide occlusal stability through proprioceptive feedback. The positioning of the occlusal contacts is primarily for static occlusion which is provided by the palatal upper buccal lower cusps (PUBL) and this occurs when we swallow. Centric

CUT VIEW

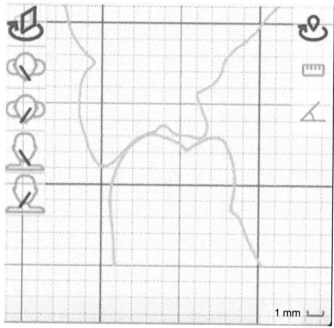

Figure 4.3   A cross-section through the cusps showing dish effect as shown on the MODJAW.

occlusion is therefore our swallowing position (hence the name habitual occlusion). From an engineering perspective, we wish to maximise the number of occlusal contacts to distribute the forces. Swallowing forces are low but repetitive so these forces can lead to microcracks; therefore the more teeth touching, the better the chance that over time the teeth will not fracture. Lear et al. (1965) have shown that swallowing contacts occur more than 1000 times a day.

The occlusal contacts should ideally be placed within the fossa or on the marginal ridge to guide the forces through the long axis because if placed on the inclines of the cusps, this can lead to fracture which may explain why cuspal fractures occur. Another reason is infraoccluded restorations because teeth have a constant eruptive force and what stops teeth from moving is an equal resistive force; this is usually from the opposing teeth but can be from soft tissues such as a tongue-thrusting habit in an anterior open bite.

Why do teeth move? To maintain proprioception. Once infraoccluded, the tooth can move or rotate to maintain proprioception and therefore change the position of the occlusal contact. Figure 4.4 highlights this.

The position of the occlusal contacts also varies according to different skeletal, molar and canine relationships.

Marginal Ridge Rule
- The lower supporting cusp when occluding with the upper tooth marginal ridge will do so with the same tooth and one tooth forward – for example, the lower second premolar

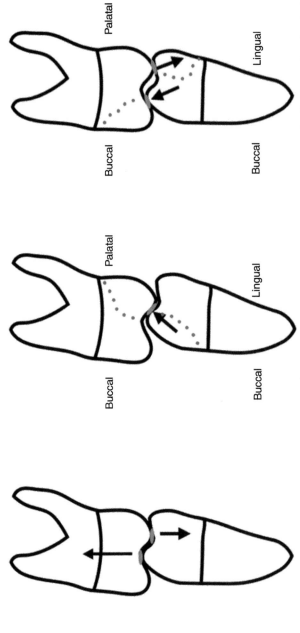

This maintains forces trajectory being placed through the long axis of the teeth and to prevent unpredictable movements and jiggling forces placed at an incline which can lead to cuspal fracture over time

Incline contacts placed in this example on the buccal incline of the palatal upper and lingual incline of the buccal lower cusp can lead to fracture of the buccal lower or palatal upper cusp

Incline contacts placed in this example on the palatal incline of the buccal upper and buccal incline of the lingual lower cusp can lead to fracture of the lingual lower or buccal upper cusp

Figure 4.4 Occlusal contacts and risks associated with incline contacts.

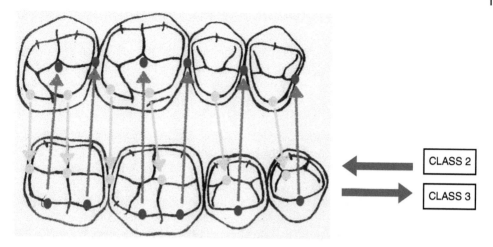

Figure 4.5 The occlusal contacts in a Class 1 relationship. The contacts then move backwards in a Class 2 and forwards in a Class 3 occlusion.

buccal (supporting) cusp will occlude with the upper second premolar mesial marginal ridge (same tooth) and the distal marginal ridge of the first premolar (one tooth forward).

- The upper supporting cusp when occluding with the lower tooth marginal ridge will do so with the same tooth and one tooth backwards – for example, the upper first molar distopalatal (supporting) cusp will occlude with the lower first molar distal marginal ridge (same tooth) and the mesial marginal ridge of the second molar (one tooth backward).

Fossa Rule
- The lower supporting cusp when contacting the upper tooth fossa will do so with same tooth only.
- The upper supporting cusp when contacting the lower tooth fossa will do so with the same tooth only (Figure 4.5).

Procedure

Survey (Visual)

The key to successful restorations is preassessing the occlusion. Equipment required to assess occlusion is as follows (please refer to Chapter 3 for description of equipment).

- *Miller's forceps* – forceps used to hold articulating paper to ensure full coverage of the teeth when marking contacts.

- *Articulating paper* – there are many thicknesses of articulating paper ranging from 8 to 200 μm. Ideally, what we require is a paper that will transfer colour easily, but this system has limitations. The challenge is interpreting the colour and the general understanding is the more colour transfer, the heavier the contact, as shown by Brizuela-Velasco (2015). However, this does not automatically translate because the force cannot be controlled so which thickness should we use? Well, the thinner the better, but why?
  - It is more precise.
  - It is conservative – you will remove less material. The example shown in Figure 4.6 shows a case and the difference in the surface area (Figure 4.6).
- *Periodontal probe* – to measure overbite and overjet. Must have millimetre graduations. UNC (University of North Carolina) 15 probes are suitable.
- *Shimstock foil* – this is 8 μm thick and is used as a holding contact and helps interpret whether the teeth are actually touching at 8 μm. Used in conjunction with articulating paper, it improves accuracy. It can be held with Miller's articulating forceps or mosquito locking forceps.
  - Step 1 – holding contact assessed on teeth adjacent to tooth being restored and contralateral side including tooth being restored.
  - Step 2 – complete restoration.
  - Step 3 – check shimstock holds as in step 1. If the restoration is high, then the restored tooth will be the only holding contact. Check with articulating paper and adjust and repeat step 1 until the same shimstock holds are achieved (Figure 4.7).

There is also occlusal wax, a modelling compound, but technology is the way forward and there are digital tools that can assist with looking at occlusal contacts such as Tekscan™ which provides information about forces, which is a limitation with articulating paper.

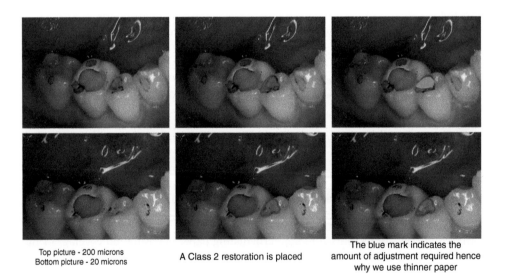

Top picture - 200 microns
Bottom picture - 20 microns

A Class 2 restoration is placed

The blue mark indicates the amount of adjustment required hence why we use thinner paper

Figure 4.6   Articulating paper difference and precision related to minimal invasiveness.

Shimstock foil - holding contacts on teeth adjacent to new restorations

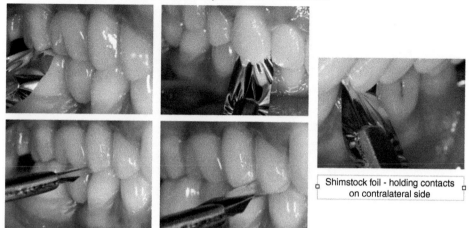

Shimstock foil - holding contacts on contralateral side

Shimstock foil - holding contacts on new restorations

Figure 4.7 Shimstock hold and how to use.

How to Transfer the Colour

The teeth must be dry – this is crucial. Place the tissue paper held in Miller's forceps and ask the patient to bite gently and hold for a few seconds. The tissue will absorb any liquid and provide a dry field. Ask the patient to tap their teeth together so the patient can rearticulate themselves, especially if they have held the mouth open for some time. This is generally done in the supine position but head and body position affect mandibular position so occlusal contacts must be checked when seated upright in the chair as well.

Then place the articulating paper over the teeth and ask the patient to close and tap their teeth together using the blue colour. This will provide static contacts. For dynamic contacts, we ask the patient to slide their teeth left and right using the red colour (ideally you want different colours for different movements). This can be difficult for patients because you are assessing the occlusion from the inside out, meaning that they are moving the jaw from a closed mouth starting point. This is an unnatural movement (unless they parafunction dynamically, i.e. bruxism) because we do not chew our food that way. To chew our food, we open our mouth and move laterally and then close, meaning outside in. So, if your patients struggle to make lateral movements, ask them to open and then move sideways and close slowly with articulating paper in between the teeth (see Figure 4.8 for example).

Fremitus (Touch)

The Survey part of the STOP process uses our eyes to assess the colour contact. Now we want to use touch to provide us with information regarding force, i.e. the greater the force, the greater the vibration (movement) of the tooth taking the force which is used for a static assessment, i.e. swallowing position. If the occlusal contact is on an incline, then this will cause a mandibular slide or deviation.

This analysis is easily performed on teeth that are more accessible, namely from premolars forward. We place our finger on the tooth – labial or buccal surface – and ask the

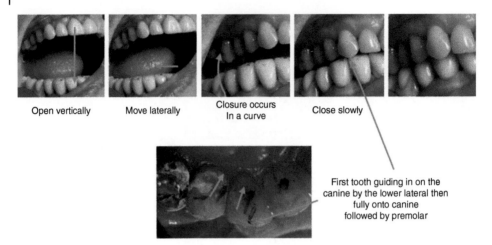

Open vertically | Move laterally | Closure occurs In a curve | Close slowly

First tooth guiding in on the canine by the lower lateral then fully onto canine followed by premolar

Figure 4.8 Dynamic occlusion assessment.

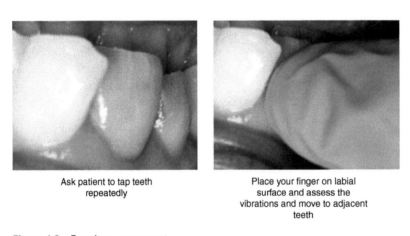

Ask patient to tap teeth repeatedly

Place your finger on labial surface and assess the vibrations and move to adjacent teeth

Figure 4.9 Fremitus assessment.

patient to tap their teeth together (Figure 4.9). If the tooth has a heavy or proud contact, it will move or vibrate more than the adjacent teeth. Move your finger to adjacent and contralateral teeth to get a good comparison. If the tooth has a heavier contact, we then use articulating paper to mark the area and adjust to lighten the force (how to adjust will be discussed in Chapter 9).

Observe (Listen)

When all the teeth meet equally, asking the patient to tap their teeth together creates a very crisp and sharp sound and this is performed before any treatment is undertaken. If the

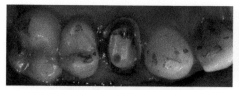

Single crown lost upper right 1st premolar
Static pre assessment - contacts on adjacent teeth

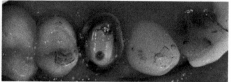

Single crown lost upper right 1st premolar
Dynamic pre assessment - group function

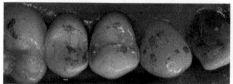

Single crown lost upper right 1st premolar
Static post assessment - contacts on adjacent teeth

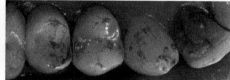

Single crown lost upper right 1st premolar
Dynamic post assessment - group function

Figure 4.10   Completion of the scenario.

restoration provided is proud, meaning that the only static contact is on this tooth, the sound changes to a dull thud-like noise. Try it for yourself by tapping your teeth together in maximum intercuspation and then move your mandible to provide only a pair of contacting teeth and tap together again and notice the difference in sound.

This is another sense we are using to assess occlusion before and after treatment. If the sound is different at the end from the start, then we use articulating paper to identify the area of supraocclusion and adjust accordingly.

Patient Feedback

This is the last step, but it is equally important; with a thorough assessment using Survey, Touch, Observe, this is an endorsement of your analysis. The first three steps are performed while the patient is supine, and our analysis must be checked with the patient sitting upright so we repeat STO before achieving our final feedback. There are still limitations to patient feedback primarily due to the use of anaesthesia and differing occlusal sensitivity thresholds. If the patient tells you something does not feel right, then please trust their judgement and recheck. The use of shimstock foil should provide some reassurance that the occlusion is right if we have equal holds in static. Figure 4.10 shows completion utilising occlusal principles discussed in the restoration of the upper right first premolar.

Conclusion

The objectives of this chapter are to:

- provide the foundations for understanding occlusion
- ensure safe practice
- conform with the patient's existing occlusion
- not ask the patient to adapt unnecessarily because this risks reorganising the occlusion unpredictably and changing the occlusal neurosignature (Figure 4.11).

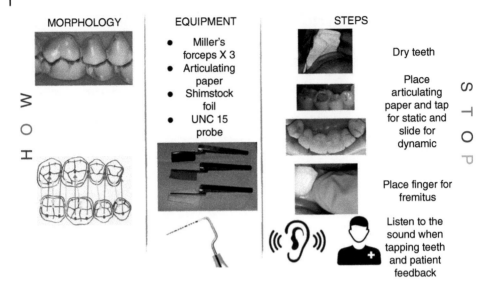

Figure 4.11 Summary of the chapter.

References

Brizuela-Velasco, A., Álvarez-Arenal, A., Ellakuria-Echevarria, J. et al. (2015). Influence of articulating paper thickness on occlusal contacts registration: a preliminary report. *Int. J. Prosthodont.* 28 (4): 360–362.

Lear, C.S., Flanagan, J.B., and Moorrees, C.F. (1965). The frequency of deglutition in man. *Arch. Oral Biol.* 10: 83–89.

Wiskott, H.W.A. and Belser, U.C. (1995). A rationale for a simplified occlusal design in restorative dentistry: historical review and clinical guidelines. *J. Prosthet. Dent.* 73 (2): 169–183.

Further Reading

Ehrlich, J. and Taicher, S. (1981). Intercuspal contacts of the natural dentition in centric occlusion. *J. Prosthet. Dent.* 45 (4): 419–421.

Korioth, T.W.P. (1990). Number and location of occlusal contacts in intercuspal position. *J. Prosthet. Dent.* 64 (2): 206–210.

5

The Crown is High

Scenario

The patient has recently had a crown placed on the upper left first molar and is not happy because his bite is different and he is uncomfortable (Figure 5.1).

Rationale

The role of teeth is to masticate food to a small enough size to swallow. Therefore, if we change the occlusion, can we safely assume we will affect mastication and swallowing and if so, how? The adaptability of the patient is also important. Some patients adapt and their chewing cycle alters mainly by reducing the width, as shown by Svensson et al. (2013) and Grigoriadis et al. (2016). However, when we look at the literature on occlusal interference studies, Clark et al. (1999) wrote a review article looking at 68 years and 18 human studies and 10 animal studies and the longest duration for which the subject had the interference was 29 days, the largest sample size was 27 subjects and the interference size was >300 μm (quite large) with a large degree of heterogeneity.

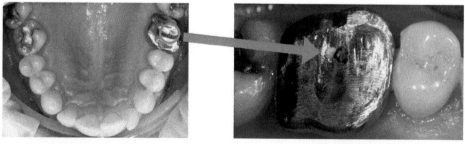

Crown fitted and then adjusted.
Patient still feeling symptoms -
pain, difficulty eating

Fossa contact from the
distobuccal cusp

Figure 5.1   Supraoccluded crown causing occlusal issues.

Practical Procedures in Dental Occlusion, First Edition. Ziad Al-Ani and Riaz Yar.
© 2022 John Wiley & Sons Ltd. Published 2022 by John Wiley & Sons Ltd.
Companion website: www.wiley.com/go/al-ani-and-riaz/dental-occlusion

Three animal studies hinted at deleterious effects to the temporomandibular joint (TMJ) and altered muscle function when the occlusal scheme was substantially disrupted but due to the length of time, they did not indicate if these changes were normal adaptations or the beginning of chronic dysfunction. The application of animal models to humans has always been an issue so the human studies looked at muscle activity using electromyographic readings of the temporalis, masseter and digastric muscles and symptoms such as pain/tenderness or clicking. In the majority of the studies, symptoms were reported with increased muscle activity and one subject in the Randow et al. (1976) study took 9 months and a stabilisation splint to alleviate the symptoms of the occlusal interference. Most subjects returned to their normal preinterference state. Within the limitations of all the studies, this tells us humans are adaptable but with different thresholds.

What are the risks of occlusal imprecision? Typically, there are three reactions when introducing something new – accept, avoid or remove.

Tooth Level

1) Pain – pulpitis.
2) Mobility – periodontitis.
3) Fracture of the tooth or restoration – or the opposing tooth.
4) Fracture or wear of other teeth – caused by altered movements to avoid the new contact; the risk is the forces now move onto other teeth – an example would be anterior tooth wear caused by forward posturing to avoid a posterior contact (overerupted wisdom tooth).
5) Migration.

Muscle Level

Pain caused by increased muscle activity and altered movements – this may be a response to removing the interference (trying to remove or avoid).

Joint Level

1) Pain caused by joint compression on the contralateral side of the proud restoration.
2) Disc displacement due to hyperactivity of the lateral pterygoid muscle (trying to remove or avoid).

The literature states that the symptoms and effects are transient but long-term studies are needed with greater standardisation of protocols and blinding to reduce bias.

If these are the reactions when the restoration is supraoccluded, this may lend itself to infraoccluding the restoration, but this is still occlusal imprecision and has short-, medium- and long-term effects.

Short-Term Risks

The forces are greater on the adjacent teeth therefore there is a risk of fracture of the adjacent teeth. This scenario is quite common among dentists when a preassessment of the

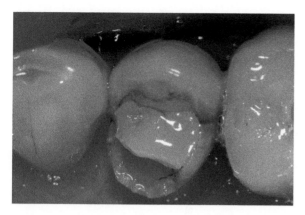

Figure 5.2   Fractured cusp following restoration of adjacent tooth with a crown.

occlusion is not performed, and a restoration is provided. In Figure 5.2 a crown was placed on the first molar 4 weeks earlier. The patient then complains that the restoration recently completed has fractured. They attend an emergency appointment and it turns out that it is the adjacent tooth that has fractured, and the patient is notified. Upon reflection, is it not possible that the dentist was the cause? There may be other causes such as caries, etc.

Medium- and Long-Term Risks

Teeth have constant eruptive force and stay in position if the opposing force is equal to the eruptive force. When there is no opposing force then teeth move until there is contact, but this is unpredictable and can lead to a change in the angulation of the forces, i.e. an incline contact and the cumulative forces over time may lead to cuspal fractures. Figure 5.3 details this progression.

Errors that lead to a proud (supraoccluded) crown include the following.

- Treatment planning stage – lack of occlusal analysis.
- Preparation stage – incorrect occlusal reduction and bite registration.
- Provisional restoration – infraoccluded provisional.
- Laboratory stage – inaccurate articulation of the model.
- Cementation stage.
- Adjustment of the restoration.

Procedure

Treatment Planning Stage

A preassessment of the occlusion helps determine whether you are conforming or reorganising. For single units, you are conforming but for multiple units or quadrant dentistry, further analysis is required.

Restorative materials are designed to take compressive forces, i.e. axially, but have poor tensile forces, i.e. non-axial forces, and guiding contacts are non-axial forces. This is not an

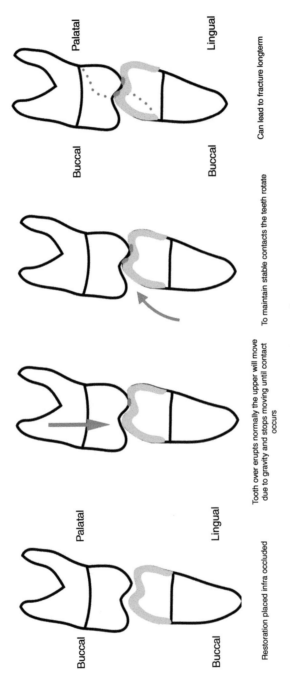

Figure 5.3 Progression of occlusal instability resulting in cuspal fracture long term.

issue if the forces are low but can cause fracture or decementation if the loads are heavy. The preassessment ensures that we provide enough bulk material thickness to withstand the load.

Occlusal Contacts – Static and Dynamic Contacts

The teeth provide guidance for the mandible and guiding teeth can be anterior or posterior. When the patient moves the mandible to the right side, this is called the working side (WS) (or laterotrusive), i.e. their chewing side. The side the mandible is moving away from is called the non-working side (NWS) (or mediotrusive).

Canine guidance is where the upper and lower canines on the WS are the only teeth in contact causing posterior teeth separation/disclusion. Physiologically, this movement is beyond functional movement because we don't want to chew with one pair of teeth.

Group function is when several pairs share the contacts on the WS (canines, premolars and molars). This is physiologically correct because you require multiple teeth to contact when chewing to break food down.

When we incise our food, we bring our mandible forward to grasp the food to bring it into the masticatory system; this movement is also called protrusive or incisional guidance (Figure 5.4).

Steele et al. (2002) stated that interferences are any tooth-to-tooth contacts that hamper or hinder smooth excursions in both static or dynamic movements. This can be on the WS or NWS and protrusive movements. Figure 5.5 shows a patient with both a NWS and WS contact or interference. The significance of interferences, particularly non-working side interference (NWSI), has been covered extensively in the literature in relation to temporo-mandibular disorder (TMD) or initiating parafunction. This is misleading as the patient in Figure 5.5 has both WS and NWS contacts, has no symptoms and has functioned like this for 50 years.

So how is this managed when providing an indirect restoration? A preassessment allows you to spot these issues following the STOP process. As a general rule, if the tooth involved is being prepared then we remove the interference, ideally at a separate appointment to allow the patient to adapt to the new excursive guidance pattern. The reason for removal before restoring with a crown is that most NWSI are on molars and the forces are greater and oblique, increasing the risk of fracture or decementation.

Steps on how to remove NWSI if providing a crown on the tooth.

1) Preassessment.
2) Identify the NWSI and assess if there are suitable teeth on the WS to take over the guidance once the interference has been removed.
3) Remove the guidance one appointment before the preparation stage.

There is another option if it is not possible to eliminate the NWSI and this involves rebuilding the WS either by adding composite material to the canine only to disclude the posterior teeth or adding material to the palatal inclines of the upper buccal cusps to provide group function on the WS. This increases the number of restorations.

Careful preassessment and postassessment will avoid the risk of introducing interferences.

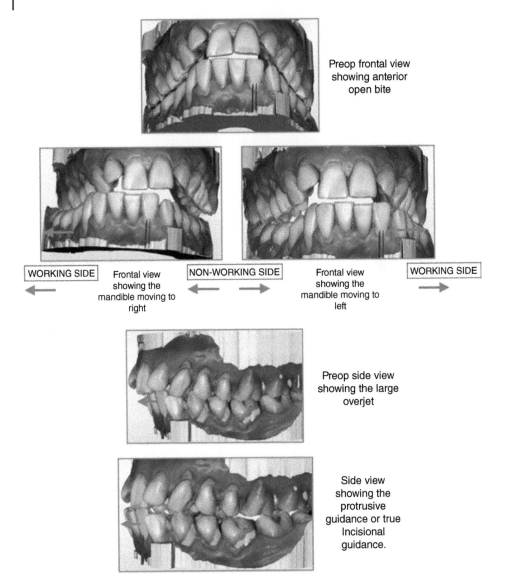

Preop frontal view showing anterior open bite

WORKING SIDE — Frontal view showing the mandible moving to right

NON-WORKING SIDE

Frontal view showing the mandible moving to left

WORKING SIDE

Preop side view showing the large overjet

Side view showing the protrusive guidance or true Incisional guidance.

Figure 5.4   Analysis of dynamic occlusion.

Preparation Stage

The restorability assessment is important before delivering a restoration because patients' expectations need to be managed. Look at:

- number of residual walls
- volume of restorations
- depth of margins (Figure 5.6).

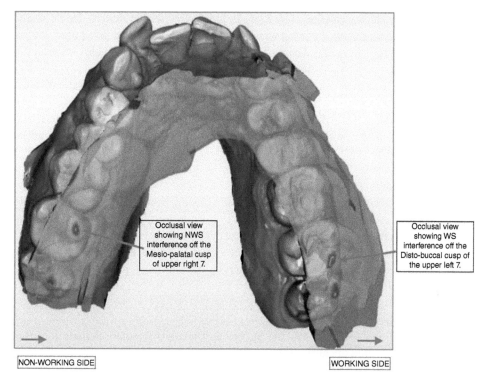

Occlusal view
showing NWS
interference off the
Mesio-palatal cusp
of upper right 7.

Occlusal view
showing WS
interference off the
Disto-buccal cusp of
the upper left 7.

NON-WORKING SIDE

WORKING SIDE

Figure 5.5   Digital scan showing WS and NWS contacts on a digital articulator.

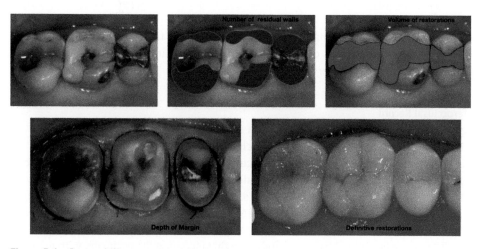

Number of residual walls

Volume of restorations

Depth of Margin

Definitive restorations

Figure 5.6   Restorability assessment in planning stage.

If you have any study casts this allows you to judge whether the models can be easily located into centric occlusion dictating whether an interocclusal record is required. It also provides an analysis of the occlusal contacts and an evaluation of the valuable interocclusal space and clinical crown height, allowing planning for margin position.

One of the most common causes of occlusal errors and supraoccluded restorations is the opposing arch impression and the impression for the provisional restoration. Meticulous impressions are essential to reduce errors that inherently occur through the process. There are three stages to ensure excellent impressions and this is equally important for the opposing arch.

Preimpression Stage

- Perforated rigid stock tray ideally (less of an issue if using heavy body silicone as opposing arch impression) and correctly extended to include the posterior teeth (use green compound). If an unusual arch shape, then use of special tray is indicated.
- Adhesive placed and allowed to set (6–8 minutes before taking impressions) or air dry otherwise adhesive acts as a lubricant and leads to the impression pulling away; this can lead to at least a 1 mm occlusal error.

Impression Seating

- Dry the teeth using tissue in Miller's forceps and gently rub some alginate into the occlusal surfaces while the nurse is loading the tray.
- Seat the tray posteriorly first and rotate upwards – this brings the material forwards and reduces gagging.
- Wait for the material to fully set (follow manufacturer's instructions).

Removal and Analysis

- When removing the tray, place fingers posteriorly on both sides and remove the tray vertically downwards – do not rotate downwards as this can cause separation of the material from the tray.
- Once removed, ensure the material has not separated from tray and remove the posterior heels if not required as this can cause distortion when seating the impression down in the disinfection bath (Figure 5.7).

Interocclusal Record

Please see Chapter 3 for occlusal registration and materials.

The interocclusal record is a record which allows mounting of the casts. Walls et al. (1991) have shown that the use of an interocclusal record can introduce inaccuracies rather than improve the articulation. The rule to adhere to is 'if the models can be easily articulated by hand, you are better with nothing at all (sometimes less is more)'. So for single units a record is generally not required. There are scenarios such as crossbites or skeletal Class 3 with reverse overjet or Class 2 with a large overjet in which the concern is that the ceramist will not be able to locate the models, so that recording the occlusion with material placed over the preparation and the adjacent teeth is the maximum required. A full arch record is required for centric relation and an arch relationship that requires stability to hold in that position such as an anterior open bite.

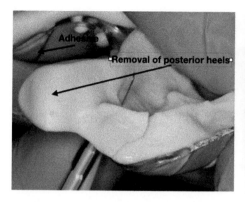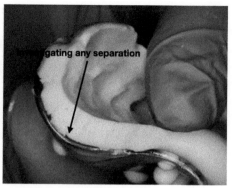

Figure 5.7   Assessment of opposing impressions to ensure no separation.

Materials available to use include the following; the key to success is how the material is used rather than the type.

- Hard wax alone.
- Hard wax as a carrier used with zinc oxide/eugenol.
- Polyvinyl siloxane.
- Acrylic resins.

Tips which will aid success.

- Use the minimum amount of material to record cusp tips or preparation.
- Avoid excess to reduce soft tissue contact and capture fissure patterns as much as possible.
- Trim record to remove undercuts (Figure 5.8).

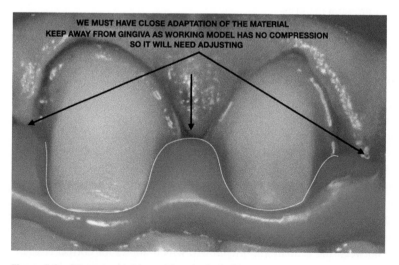

Figure 5.8   Bite record taking with polyvinyl siloxane.

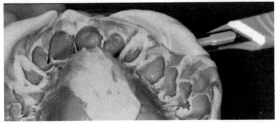
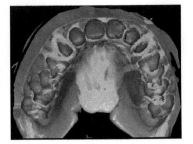

Trimming silicone to facilitate removal from stone cast

Figure 5.9   Trimming silicone to aid study cast fabrication.

Verification of the Study Models

A final step to ensure that the study models accurately replicate the intraoral occlusal situation is to hold the casts tightly together and determine if the shimstock holds are the same as they are in the mouth.

Before sending the impressions to the laboratory for casting and fabrication, a helpful tip which will endear you to the ceramist is to trim the outer excess material and undercuts to facilitate removal of the silicone/alginate after casting. This will reduce occlusal errors and improve accuracy (Figure 5.9).

Laboratory Stage

Regardless of the impression material or the laboratory technique employed, it is not possible to have an exact duplicate of the mouth. The reasons are that the model is solid and the patient's arch has a periodontal ligament and the mandible and maxilla are elastic – it was shown by Gates and Nicholls (1981) that the mandible decreases in width by 0.5 mm at the second molar level when opening and moving protrusively. Other reasons for differences are discussed by Linke et al. (1985):

- distortion of the impression material
- stone expansion
- defects on the occlusal surfaces
- distortion of the interocclusal record
- insufficient adaptation of the intermaxillary registration.

Ways to improve accuracy include casting the models as soon as possible if using alginate and trimming models to remove 'blobs' created by air holes in the impressions. If an interocclusal record is provided, this is trimmed to allow for full seating on the model and articulation with the opposing model. Careful handling at this stage will reduce occlusal errors. Additional information regarding occlusion improves occlusal accuracy. This can be obtained using shimstock holds or photographs showing occlusal contacts detailing the thickness of articulating paper used. This allows the ceramist to verify that the contacts on the model match those in the mouth.

When fabricating the crown, a die spacer is used with the objective of reducing the hydraulic pressure between the cement and the crown, which allows for correct seating and for excess cement to escape, reducing occlusal errors. The ideal die spacer should be between 25 and 40 μm according to McLean and von Fraunhofer (1971).

Articulator

A small number of restorations that are not involved in excursions can be done on a simple hinge articulator and the restoration adjusted in situ. Crowns involved in excursive movements require an articulator that has similar anatomical dimensions, but the reality is they do not exist. The best articulator is the human. Static contacts can be accurately delivered if the models have the same arc of closure but dynamic contacts are difficult to replicate because the ball joint of the articulator is spherical while the human condylar head is oval, the mechanical glenoid fossa of the articulator is angular with fixed and solid dimensions (i.e. no disc) yet the human glenoid fossa has a bony border with a cartilage disc.

Provisional Restoration

This stage is often rushed and treated as an afterthought. This is a very important step in ensuring that the teeth do not move, thus introducing further errors at cementation stage.

The objectives of a provisional restoration are to:

- maintain occlusal relationship
- protect pulp and gingival architecture
- maintain mesiodistal proportions
- test aesthetics and occlusion
- check thickness
- check parellelism of preps when fabricating a bridge.

A preassessment of the occlusion allows the clinician to maintain the adjacent occlusal contacts and introduce further occlusal contacts on the provisional restoration.

The provisional restoration materials most commonly used are

Polymethyl methacylate acrylic (PMMA) and bisacryl composite resins. Both have advantages and disadvantages – the key is to use the material correctly and to ensure a stable occlusion (Figure 5.10).

When adjusting the occlusion of the provisional restoration, the bulk of the adjustment may be completed with the patient in supine position, but must be finished with the patient sitting upright. Posture will affect mandibular position and the patient doesn't chew their food when lying down!

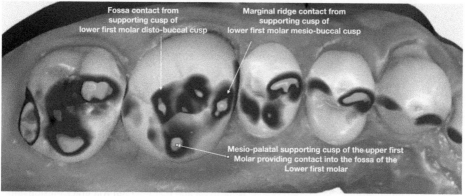

Provisional restoration designed to maintain occlusal contacts of adjacent teeth
And occlusal stability of the restoration

Fossa contact from supporting cusp of lower first molar disto-buccal cusp

Marginal ridge contact from supporting cusp of lower first molar mesio-buccal cusp

Mesio-palatal supporting cusp of the upper first Molar providing contact into the fossa of the Lower first molar

Figure 5.10 Digital design of provisional crown.

(a) (b) (c)

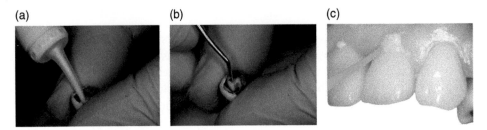

Figure 5.11 (a–c) Cementation of a crown.

Cementation Stage

If the die spacer is between 25 and 40 µm, that means we do not need a lot for cement to be placed. Remove the provisional restoration. Check the occlusal contacts on the adjacent teeth and opposing arch with shimstock and articulating paper so you have the baseline recorded. Try the restoration in and recheck. If the shimstock is not holding on the adjacent teeth, then the restoration is supraoccluded. Using articulating paper, mark the proud contact and adjust until contact and the shimstock holds on the adjacent teeth are the same as the baseline. If the crown is infraoccluded then it can be sent back to the laboratory for additional porcelain to be added. Once adjusted, polish with the correct polishing burs for porcelain.

Tips for cementing crowns.

- Fill the base of the crown to approximately a third of the crown height (Figure 5.11a).
- Using a flat plastic smear the cement on the walls of the restoration (Figure 5.11b).
- Seat the restoration and remove excess using a microbrush (Figure 5.11c).

Scenario Completion

Figure 5.12 showing completion of the provisional restoration with stable static contacts and shimstock holds. At subsequent 8 week review patient symptoms had disappeared.

(a)

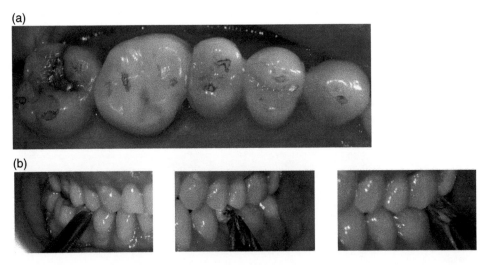

(b)

Figure 5.12 (a) Provisional restoration seated. Note fossa and marginal ridge contact. Mesiopalatal cusp providing occlusal contact. (b) Shim stock holds on adjacent and restored tooth including contralateral side.

References

Clark, G.T., Tsukiyama, Y., Baba, K., and Watanabe, T. (1999). Sixty eight years of experimental occlusal interference studies: what have we learned? *J. Prosthet. Dent.* 82: 704–713.

Gates, G.N. and Nicholls, J.I. (1981). Evaluation of mandibular arch width change. *J. Prosthet. Dent.* 46: 385–392.

Grigoriadis, J., Trulsson, M., and Svensson, K. (2016). Motor behavior during the first chewing cycle in subjects with fixed tooth or implant supported prostheses. *Clin. Oral Implants Res.* 27: 473–480.

Linke, B., Nicholls, J.I., and Faucher, R. (1985). Distortion analysis of stone casts made from impression materials. *J. Prosthet. Dent.* 54: 794–802.

McLean, J.W. and von Fraunhofer, J.A. (1971). The estimation of cement film thickness by an in vivo; technique. *Br. Dent. J.* 131: 107–111.

Randow, K., Carlsson, K., Edlund, J., and Oberg, T. (1976). The effect of an occlusal interference on the masticatory system. An experimental investigation. *Odontol. Rev.* 27: 245–256.

Steele, J.G., Nohl, F.S.A., and Wassell, R.W. (2002). Crowns and other extra-coronal restorations: occlusal considerations and articulator selection. *Br. Dent. J.* 192 (7): 377–380.

Svensson, K., Grigoriades, J., and Trulsson, M. (2013). Alterations in intra-oral manipulation and splitting of food by subjects with tooth or implant-supported fixed prostheses. *Clin. Oral Implants Res.* 24: 549–555.

Walls, A.W.G., Wassell, R.W., and Steele, J.G. (1991). A comparison of two methods for locating the intercuspal position (ICP) whilst mounting casts on an articulator. *J. Oral Rehabil.* 18: 43–48.

6

My Bite Feels Different

A patient attends complaining of pain over the right side of his face in front of his ear, headache and a feeling of restricted jaw movement 3 days after he had a fixed-movable bridge fitted to replace a missing upper right first premolar tooth. Following the provision of the bridge, he said that his 'bite felt different' and he returned to see his dentist for this problem (Figure 6.1).

What was the Most Likely Cause of the Patient's Complaint?

A bridge made without careful consideration of the patient's occlusion is potentially hazardous. When a tooth in an arch is prepared for an indirect restoration, it is necessary to ensure that an accurate occlusal record is transmitted to your technician.

A functionally stable posterior occlusion exists when enough teeth are in simultaneous even contact and occlusal forces are directed axially, thereby stabilising the position not only of the teeth but also of the temporomandibular joints (TMJs). Appropriate occlusal stability distributes occlusal forces over a wide area, preventing damage to the individual components of the masticatory system. The way to achieve this is to adopt a conformative approach, which is defined as the provision of restorations 'in harmony with the existing jaw relationships'. In practice, this means that the occlusion of the new restoration is

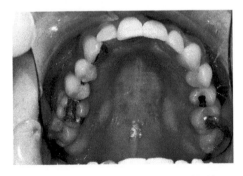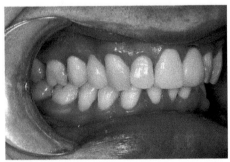

Figure 6.1   Intraoral view of the fitted bridge.

Practical Procedures in Dental Occlusion, First Edition. Ziad Al-Ani and Riaz Yar.
© 2022 John Wiley & Sons Ltd. Published 2022 by John Wiley & Sons Ltd.
Companion website: www.wiley.com/go/al-ani-and-riaz/dental-occlusion

provided in such a way that the occlusal contacts of other teeth remain unaltered. The reason why this approach is favoured is not because it is the easiest but because it is the safest. It is less likely to introduce potentially harmful consequences for the tooth, periodontium, muscles, TMJ, patient and dentist!

The dentist must understand how all the interrelated parts of the total masticatory system work in harmony and if any one part of the system gets out of harmony, all the other parts are affected.

Ignoring the conformative approach may result in a less than ideal occlusion that is not harmonious with the existing occlusion, and the patient may not tolerate this. The occlusion of the bridge that had been provided for the patient was obviously not the same as he had had pretreatment and he developed a temporomandibular disorder (TMD) almost immediately after this bridge was fitted.

What is notable in this patient is that, when the occlusion was restored to the original, the symptoms disappeared rapidly. This depends on the timescale for placement of the iatrogenically introduced occlusal interference. The sooner that it is removed, the quicker the symptoms will disappear.

How Can This Conformative Approach Be Adopted Practically?

The patient's occlusion should be recorded before any treatment is started. The construction of an indirect restoration requires the transfer of anatomical information from the clinician to the dental laboratory technician. This requires accurate models of the patient's teeth and an occlusal record, a centric jaw relation and a facebow record. Bite registration paste is better than a wax occlusal registration (see Chapter 3).

It is essential to have a good record of the patient's occlusion if any treatment is to be provided that may have the potential for changing the occlusion. This record provides a benchmark against which the patient's occlusal pattern can be compared. Moreover, occlusal records are essential for medicolegal reasons.

Ideally, before tooth preparation is undertaken, occlusal contacts should be checked with articulating paper and shimstock (Figure 6.2), not only on the teeth to be prepared but also on the adjacent teeth. A record should be made of the occlusal contacts. Unless the models exhibit exactly the same occlusal contacts as the patient's teeth, the likelihood is that the dentist will find that 'the bite is wrong' on the restoration at the fit stage. This is a not unfamiliar scenario and care at this stage will minimise, although not eliminate, the chance of error. To prevent the restoration being made on models with an inaccurate occlusion, it is important to adopt a means of checking the patient's occlusion as well as the occlusion of the models before starting the laboratory process.

An occlusal examination should record whether or not centric relation/retruded contact position CR/RCP (Figure 6.3) and centric occlusion/intercuspal position CO/ICP, the habitual bite, are coincident. If not, where is the premature contact and is there a slide from CR to the habitual bite CO? If there is a slide, is it a large or small slide, is it in the same sagittal plane or is it off to one side or the other? Is there anterior guidance on the canine teeth, which is the ideal, and are there any working or non-working side interferences up

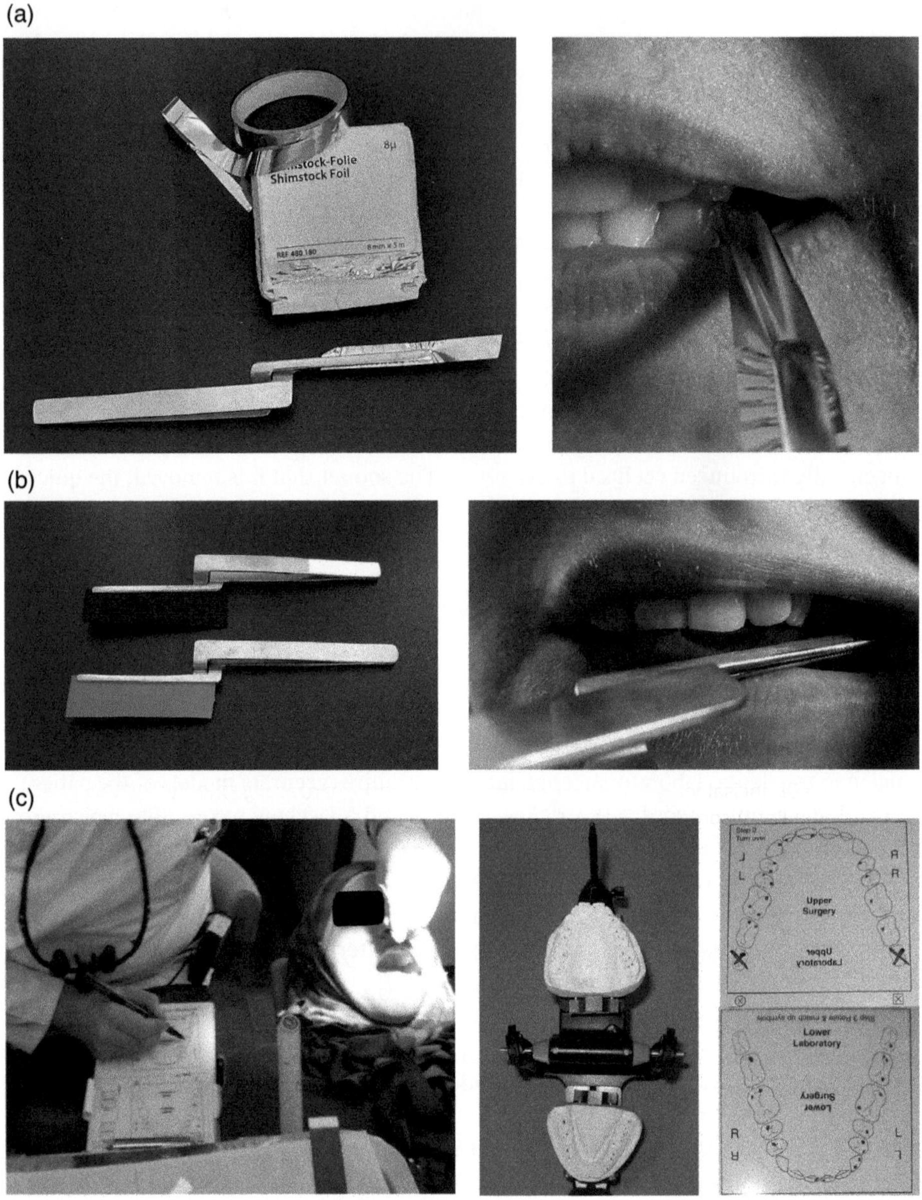

(a)

(b)

(c)

Figure 6.2 (a) Shimstock is 8 μm thick metal foil used as a feeler gauge between occluding teeth. (b) Articulating papers held with Miller's forceps to mark occlusal contacts. (c) Recording the patient's static and dynamic occlusal contacts at the chairside. *Source:* Al-Ani Z, Gray RJM. (2021). Temporomandibular Disorders: A Problem-Based Approach, 2nd edn. John Wiley & Sons Ltd, Chichester.

to and beyond the canine crossover position? These features should be recorded to enable the dentist to adhere to a conformative approach when performing restorative treatment and to have a baseline for later comparison.

It is important for the dentist to record whether there is freedom in centric occlusion. This is especially important when restoring anterior teeth with, for instance, crowns, as any

(a)

(b)

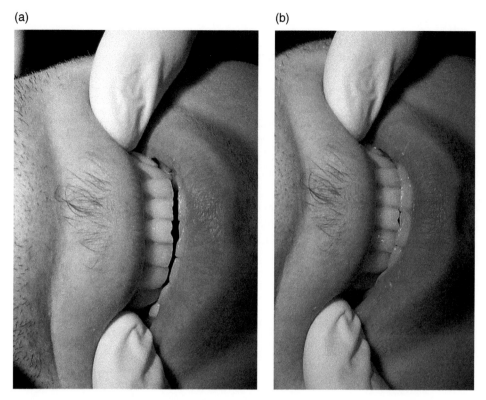

Figure 6.3 (a) CR incisal view and (b) CO incisal view. *Source:* Al-Ani Z, Gray RJM. (2021). Temporomandibular Disorders: A Problem-Based Approach, 2nd edn. John Wiley & Sons Ltd, Chichester.

retrusion of the mandible by placing restorations that are thicker than the teeth were originally could cause immediate TMD symptoms or trauma to the restored teeth due to the mandible being forced distally.

Can the Dentist Adjust the Teeth Opposing the Bridge to Improve the Occlusion and Hopefully Reduce the Patient's Discomfort? No!

This is obviously wrong and is medicolegally indefensible. It was apparent that a change in the patient's occlusion was caused by placement of the permanent bridge to an incorrect occlusion, and this was directly responsible for the onset of the TMD symptoms. This was further reinforced by the fact that, when the occlusion was corrected by placement and subsequent adjustment of the temporary bridge, the symptoms resolved rapidly.

A provisional bridge was made, and the patient's symptoms resolved. A final permanent restoration was constructed and he remained symptom free.

Further Reading

Al-Ani, Z. (2020). Occlusion and Temporomandibular Disorders: A Long-Standing Controversy in Dentistry. *Primary Dent. J.* 9: 43–48.

Alani, A. and Patel, M. (2014). Clinical issues in occlusion – Part I. *Singapore Dent. J.* 35C: 31–38.

Burke, F.J., Murray, M.C., and Shortall, A.C. (2005). Trends in indirect dentistry: 6. Provisional restorations, more than just a temporary. *Dent. Update* 32: 443–452.

Davies, S. (2004). Conformative, re-organized or unorganized? *Dent. Update* 31: 334–345.

Davies, S.J., Gray, R.M., and Smith, P.W. (2001). Good occlusal practice in simple restorative dentistry. *Br. Dent. J.* 191: 365–381.

Patel, M. and Alani, A. (2015). Clinical issues in occlusion – Part II. *Singapore Dent. J.* 36: 2–11.

Shargill, I. and Ashley, M. (2006). Good night, squashbite: a 'how to' paper on better wax occlusal records. *Dent. Update* 33: 626–631.

7

'My Front Tooth Filling Keeps Fracturing'

Scenario

A patient attends complaining of a repeated fracturing of his upper left central incisor. This has occurred three times in a period of 5 months. He is embarrassed by the aesthetics and would like a restoration that lasts longer. He has been recommended that the tooth be 'crowned' (Figure 7.1).

Rationale

The anterior teeth are crucial for function. The central incisors (and first permanent molars) are the first teeth to erupt and establish the chewing motion within the central pattern generators. The proprioception on the anterior teeth is greater because this information is required to deliver the forces via the muscles to break the food down. The central incisor is also crucial for phonetics and aesthetics and this will also be addressed in this chapter (Figure 7.2).

A common problem that presents is the chipping of anterior restorations provided because the teeth are wearing. One-off incidents such as assault, fall, opening objects with the teeth, etc. are not discussed here.

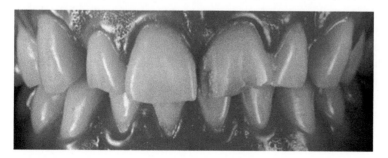

Figure 7.1

Practical Procedures in Dental Occlusion, First Edition. Ziad Al-Ani and Riaz Yar.
© 2022 John Wiley & Sons Ltd. Published 2022 by John Wiley & Sons Ltd.
Companion website: www.wiley.com/go/al-ani-and-riaz/dental-occlusion

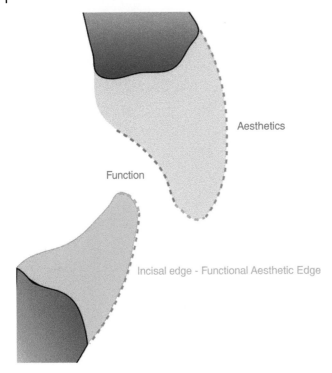

Aesthetics

Function

Incisal edge - Functional Aesthetic Edge

Figure 7.2   The important aspects of the incisors and their role.

Procedure

A careful occlusal assessment involves a static and dynamic analysis.

Static Assessment

- *Incisal relationship* – this indicates the force trajectory when either biting into food (physiology) or parafunction/hypernormal function (pathology) (Figure 7.3).
- *Overbite* – this is the vertical overlap of the incisors and is related to the skeletal and incisal relationship. Measured in millimetres or as a percentage of overlap of the mandibular incisor. Measured using a periodontal probe – UNC 15.
- *Overjet* – this is the horizontal overlap of the incisor and is related to the skeletal and incisal relationship. A common measuring error is the starting reference point which is the palatal margin of the incisal edge not the labial margin because you are then including the incisal edge thickness in your measurement. Measured in millimetres (Figure 7.4).

Dynamic Assessment

- *Incisional or protrusive guidance* – this is the mandibular movement required to incise and involves opening and bringing the mandible forward and closing until the food is grasped (Figure 7.5). This is a physiological movement and occurs *outside–in*. Another

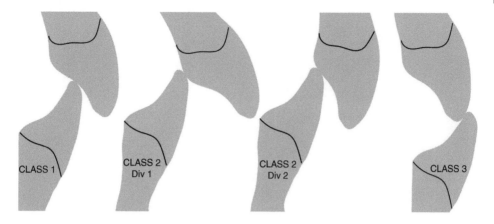

- Class I – the lower incisor edges occlude with or lie immediately below the cingulum plateau of the upper central incisors.

- Class II – the lower incisor edges lie posterior to the cingulum plateau. There are two subdivisions of this

    - Division 1 – the upper central incisors are proclined or of average inclination and there is an increase in overjet.

    - Division 2 – The upper central incisors are retroclined. The overjet is usually minimal or may be increased.

- Class III – The lower incisor edges lie anterior to the cingulum plateau of the upper incisors. The overjet is reduced or reversed.

Figure 7.3   Incisal relationships.

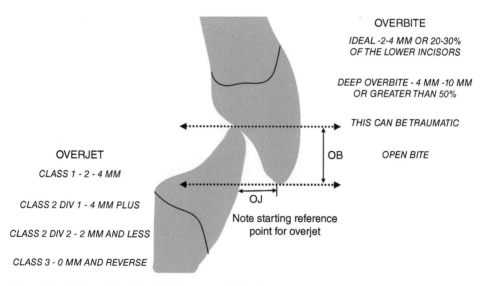

Figure 7.4   Horizontal and vertical overlap of the incisors.

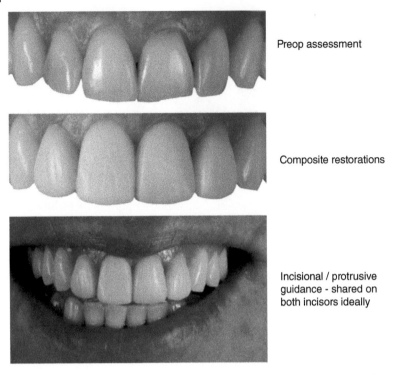

Preop assessment

Composite restorations

Incisional / protrusive
guidance - shared on
both incisors ideally

Figure 7.5   Anterior composites and occlusal design when incising or protrusive movement.

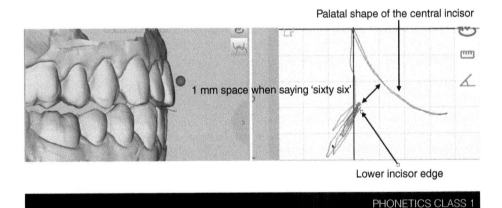

Palatal shape of the central incisor

1 mm space when saying 'sixty six'

Lower incisor edge

PHONETICS CLASS 1

Figure 7.6   Phonetics in a Class 1 incisal relationship.

method is to ask the patient to slide the jaw forward with the teeth together; this is
inside–out and is an unnatural movement unless they have habits or parafunction that
way. Both movements need assessing but more importantly when wear is present. The
objective is to share the forces between both central incisors.

- *Phonetics* (Figure 7.6) – a very important aspect which is usually not given the necessary
  consideration. Silverman (1951) used phonetics to assess vertical dimension and Fradeani
  (2004) stressed the importance of this when aesthetically rehabilitating his patients.

Articulation of speech is a complex pathway, as discussed in Chapter 2. The articulation of speech (Elsubeihi et al. 2019) involves active and passive articulators.

- Active articulators – carry out all or most of the movement during speech. These are the lower lip, tongue and the mandible with the lower incisors.
- Passive articulators – the articulators that make little or no movement during speech. These are the upper lip, maxillary teeth and posterior pharynx.

The human smile has many components; the central incisors are crucial and the use of letters/words is important in aiding display of the central incisors. Ideally, this needs to be recorded on a video of the patient or by taking photographs. The initial analysis regarding central incisors is the visibility at rest. The amount visible is approximately 2.0 mm for males and 3.5 mm for females and this decreases with age due to wear and loss of muscle tone (Vig and Brundo 1978). The smile line is another important element that must be evaluated, and this depends upon the mobility of the upper lip.

Letters and words that aid the process of assessment include the following.

- 'M' or 'EMMA' – method for assessing maxillary central incisors at rest.
- 'E' or 'EEEEEEEE' – method for assessing maxillary central incisors when smiling.
- 'F' or 'V' – method used to analyse maxillary central incisor position in regard to the lower lip, i.e. length and anterior–posterior positioning. 'F' is on the vermillion border and 'V' is inside the vermillion border.
- 'S' or 'Sixty-six' – method used to analyse maxillary central incisor edge position with an ideal space of 1–1.5 mm between the incisal edges of the anterior teeth during pronunciation (Pound 1977). Excessive space can lead to lisping.

The use of phonetics in assessing occlusal vertical dimension (OVD) will be addressed later in the book.

Cause of Wear

The first issue when aiming to restore front teeth is to understand the cause of the wear, and whether this is trauma related. Common causes include the following.

- *Hypernormal function* – nail biting (Figure 7.7) or placement of external objects that act as a habit such as pen biting, hair clips, coffee stirrers, etc. The cumulative habit over a lifetime will cause microcracks and can lead to potential loss of the tooth. Making the patient aware of this usually leads to a change in habits.
- *Skeletal management* – Class 3 incisal edge relationships. These cases require either orthodontics to correct the interincisal relationship or a careful conformative approach to restorations (Figure 7.8). An understanding of the patient's desires means simple treatments can deliver effective results.
- *Deflective contact posteriorly causing anterior thrust* – the first tooth contact on a posterior tooth can cause the mandible to deviate off this contact and anteriorly thrust, leading to constant trauma with chipping and anterior tooth wear.

The case described below requires a careful history and assessment. The most common cause is an overerupted third molar which means that centric occlusion (CO) is not stable because of the mandibular deviation to avoid this tooth or the introduction of an interference by providing a restoration.

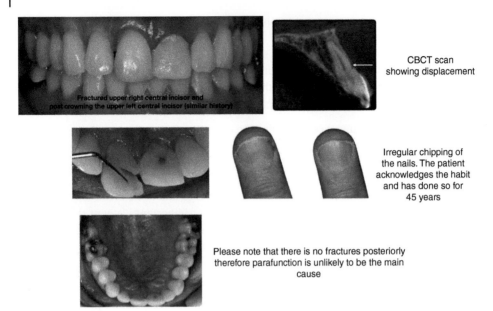

Fractured upper right central incisor and post crowning the upper left central incisor (similar history)

CBCT scan showing displacement

Irregular chipping of the nails. The patient acknowledges the habit and has done so for 45 years

Please note that there is no fractures posteriorly therefore parafunction is unlikely to be the main cause

Figure 7.7 Fracture resulting from a nail-biting habit (hypernormal function).

The reference position to utilise is centric relation – see Chapter 3 for techniques.

The first tooth contact when the condyles are seated in the glenoid fossa is the centric relation contact position (CRCP). The case shown in Figure 7.8 details such a scenario. The patient initially received a traumatic blow while at work which resulted in fracturing of upper left 1. This was repaired using composite. This initial restoration lasted 2 weeks so it was repeated; it failed again at 6 weeks, was replaced again, and the restoration was lost again 8 weeks later. The patient then sought a second opinion. The management and assessment are shown in Figure 7.9.

(a)

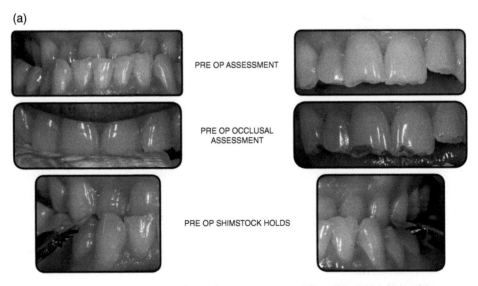

PRE OP ASSESSMENT

PRE OP OCCLUSAL ASSESSMENT

PRE OP SHIMSTOCK HOLDS

Figure 7.8 (a, b) A case showing conformative management of Class 3 incisal relationship.

(b)

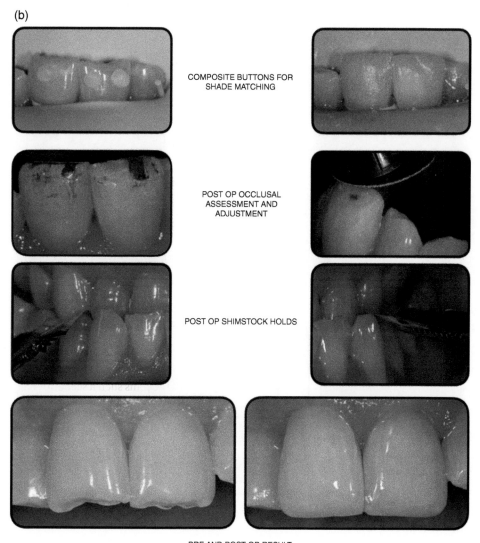

COMPOSITE BUTTONS FOR
SHADE MATCHING

POST OP OCCLUSAL
ASSESSMENT AND
ADJUSTMENT

POST OP SHIMSTOCK HOLDS

PRE AND POST OP RESULT

Figure 7.8 (Cont'd)

The mandible then slides down the cuspal slopes into centric occlusion. The movement of the mandible will have a minimum of two passages, and this depends upon the point on the cusp at which the tooth contacts, i.e. if it is on an incline or cusp tip (Figure 7.10).

The treatment in this case is to remove the upper left 8 as it is unopposed and creating disharmony and then restore the upper left central incisor. The question is where does the CRCP move too then? It will move to another tooth posteriorly – the original tooth that was in contact before the upper left 8 overerupted. Before you restore, assess the occlusion in static and dynamic. The static contact needs to be contacting either the restoration or the tooth, *not* the restoration interface. Dynamic contact ideally should be placed on the tooth; if this is not possible, then contact should be placed on the restoration, but the restoration requires more bulk to withstand the tensile forces.

(a)

Fractured upper left central incisor
caused initially by trauma
but the restoration is not staying insitu
for longer than 2 months at a time

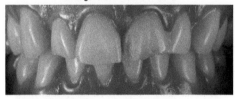

Centric Occlusion

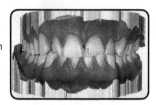

Green compound acting as
anterior deprogrammer/bite platform

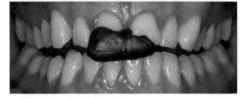

Centric Relation
Contact Position

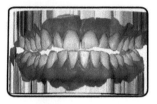

(b)

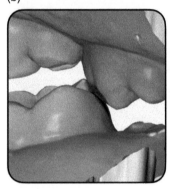
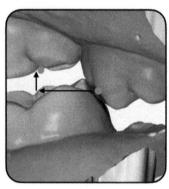

Slide from CRCP to CO

This can be either
1. Horizontal
2. Vertical
3. Lateral

In this case we have a
Large Horizontal
And small Vertical component to the
Slide
THIS HORIZONTAL MOVEMENT
IS THE THRUST THAT CAN CAUSE
ANTERIOR WEAR

Figure 7.9   (a) Preoperative assessment. (b) CRCP-CO slide resulting in a forward thrust – deflective contact.

(c)

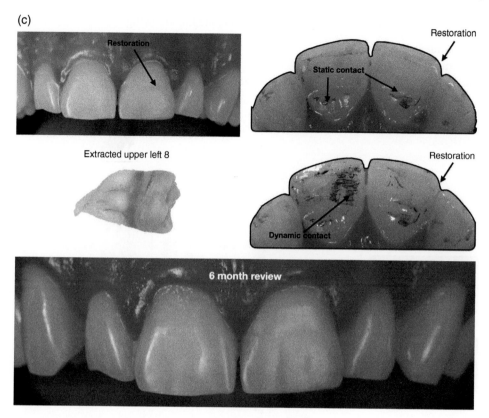

Figure 7.9 (Cont'd)   (c) Final restoration with occlusal design.

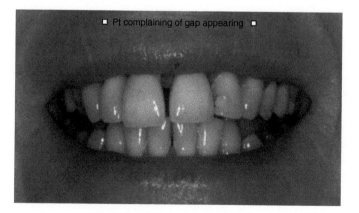

Figure 7.10   Migration resulting from deflective contact.

Signs that this deflective contact is a problem include the following.

- Continued chipping.
- Fremitus – mobility.
- Migration – tooth movement with no periodontal pocketing noted (Figure 7.10).

Summary

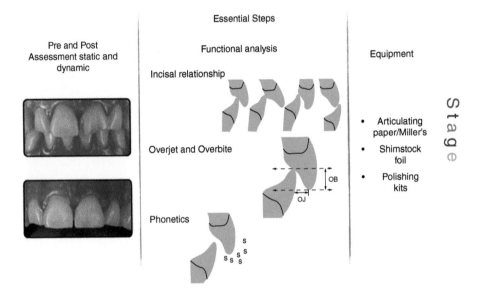

Figure 7.11   Summary of the chapter.

References

Elsubeihi, E.S., Elkareimi, Y., and Elbishari, H. (2019). Phonetic considerations in restorative dentistry. *Dent. Update* 46: 880–893.

Fradeani, M. (2004). Esthetic Rehabilitation in Fixed Prosthodontics, vol. 1, 117–134. Chicago: Quintessence.

Pound, E. (1977). Let/S/be your guide. *J. Prosthet. Dent.* 38: 482–489.

Silverman, M.M. (1951). Accurate measurement of vertical dimension by phonetics and the speaking centric space. Part 1. *Dent. Dig.* 57: 261–265.

Vig, R.G. and Brundo, G.C. (1978). The kinetics of anterior tooth display. *J. Prosthet. Dent.* 39: 502–504.

8

TMD and Occlusion – Is There a Link?

A relatively new patient, Mrs Smith, a 43-year-old housewife, has come to see you because of pain in her face. The pain is associated with the area in front of her ear. It is mainly on the left-hand side but can occur on the right as well.

The pain is worse in the morning and at the end of the day. It also gets painful when she eats some meals and sometimes, she will wake because of the pain. She has visited her dentist in the past who investigated her teeth and found no dental pathology. She has had a click in this jaw for the last 3 years and occasionally feels her opening is limited but can open here mouth fully.

Here opening comment was :'I have researched it on the internet and I know what needs to be done . . . my bite needs to be adjusted!'.

Is There Any Evidence to Support the Use of Occlusal Adjustment as an Initial Therapy in TMD Management?

Opinion regarding the importance of occlusion as an aetiological factor in the development of temporomandibular disorders (TMDs) has shifted between it being the main causative factor and there being no correlation at all. Some authors believe that occlusion is the primary factor in the onset of TMD symptoms, whereas others feel that occlusion has no role and that aetiological factors are based more on behavioural, psychological and neurological problems.

Moreover, the relationship between TMD and malocclusion also remains controversial, but there is no evidence to support an increased incidence of TMD in patients with malocclusion.

To date, most occlusal studies have assessed the static relationship of the teeth and considered the significance, or non-significance, of occlusal factors in relation to TMDs only when signs and symptoms are present. The findings are certainly not conclusive regarding any single factor being consistently associated with a TMD.

Many experimental, epidemiological and clinical studies have failed to support a significant role of occlusion in the development of a TMD as the remodelling capacity of the articulatory system would allow accommodation to most occlusal functions and

Practical Procedures in Dental Occlusion, First Edition. Ziad Al-Ani and Riaz Yar.
© 2022 John Wiley & Sons Ltd. Published 2022 by John Wiley & Sons Ltd.
Companion website: www.wiley.com/go/al-ani-and-riaz/dental-occlusion

dysfunctions. It is a biological system which is able to adapt to various morphological features until stability is achieved. Some occlusal features, however, may place greater adaptive demands on the system. While most individuals compensate without problems, adaptation in others may lead to greater risk of dysfunction.

Furthermore, controlled studies of occlusal factors and TMD show either no relationship or at best only a weak correlation between specific variables and TMD.

Many authors concluded that many occlusal parameters, traditionally believed to be influential, contribute only in a minor manner to the development of TMDs and that the occlusion cannot be considered to be the most important factor in the aetiology of a TMD.

It has been suggested that some occlusal variables may be a result rather than a cause of TMD.

A recent systematic review reviewed the literature on the association between features of dental occlusion and TMDs. It concluded that, although there were a few papers that may have suggested a possible association, the existing evidence supports the absence of a disease-specific association, and there is no reason to hypothesise a major role for dental occlusion in the pathophysiology of TMDs. The authors recommended that dental clinicians will need to move towards acceptance of the biopsychosocial model and abandon some of the older beliefs about treating TMD.

As mentioned earlier, much of the basis for the idea that 'occlusion' plays a major role in the aetiology of TMD comes from observing the results of various occlusal therapies, and many of the theories which support the association are unsubstantiated.

Occlusal Adjustment for Treating TMD Patients

Occlusal adjustments may be tempting to the clinician. If there is obvious interference, in the past it has been suggested that 'picking up a handpiece and removing the interference' may lead to an improvement in the patient's TMD symptoms. This, however, is a dangerous course of action if previous analysis of articulated and mounted study casts and a plaster equilibration have not been undertaken. Otherwise, removal of premature contacts or interferences will be merely guesswork. It is similar to the analogy of sawing the legs off a table without any measurement. If a part is removed from one leg, it is frequently necessary to form repeated adjustments to the other three legs until a stable position is reached, if indeed this can be achieved.

A Cochrane systematic review reported that there was no evidence from randomised controlled trials (RCTs) that occlusal adjustments prevent or manage a TMD and, therefore, occlusal adjustment cannot be recommended for the management or prevention of TMD.

It is apparent when treating a patient with an occlusally balanced appliance that the mandibular position can alter quite markedly as treatment progresses and painful muscles relax. For this reason, what initially might be deemed to be an occlusal interference or premature contact at the onset of treatment might not be one at the end.

Moreover, as an initial therapy, occlusal adjustment is not recommended as jaw and tooth relationships cannot be accurately determined in the presence of pain. The approach of 'pick up a handpiece and remove interferences at the first visit' is not defensible.

It would therefore appear to be sound advice not to make permanent and irreversible adjustments to the occlusion in the presence of a TMD, as when the disc is repositioned occlusal contacts will change. Some occlusal variables, therefore, may be a result rather than a cause of TMD.

Caution should be exercised in the use of occlusal adjustment as a remedy for TMD, as this can cause medicolegal concerns. Medicolegally, it is difficult to defend haphazard removal of tooth substance or the surface of crowns or other restorations in an attempt to treat a TMD if this has not been preplanned, and it should therefore be avoided.

There is insufficient evidence to suggest that any occlusal treatment is as effective, or more effective, than any other rehabilitation treatment in TMD.

There is also insufficient evidence to support the generalised preventive influence of occlusal adjustment or orthodontic correction of malocclusion on TMD development.

In general, the evidence reviewed was not supportive of occlusal adjustment as therapy for TMD and the literature suggests that occlusal equilibration should not be provided as an initial therapy for TMD patients, and should not be performed to prevent or treat signs or symptoms.

It has also been suggested that if an anterior repositioning appliance successfully treats symptoms of an internal derangement, then the occlusion should be restored to the treatment position. Contrary to what some practitioners advocate, however, occlusal therapy is not needed to maintain a TMD patient's long-term symptomatic improvement.

Since occlusal treatments are typically irreversible and the evidence of their therapeutic or preventive effects on TMD is insufficient, it is recommended that reversible treatment such as self-care, well-designed splints, physiotherapy and pharmacotherapy should always be used initially to manage signs and symptoms of TMD. As symptoms of pain and dysfunction in a TMD patient may come and go without any obvious change in any recognisable factor, one must be very hesitant about introducing any permanent changes in any part of the gnathological system.

Irreversible occlusal adjustments should never be undertaken in the presence of acute muscle pain or TMD symptoms. Ideally, occlusal adjustments should not be done until after a period of successful splint treatment. If a well-balanced stabilisation splint is worn and the patient's symptoms resolve, only to return when the splint is 'weaned off', then there might be a logical reason to address the occlusion of the natural teeth, but not without further detailed occlusal analysis, and only after meticulous planning with articulated plaster casts and with informed and valid consent. This would indicate whether provision of an 'improved' occlusion would benefit the patient's symptoms.

If occlusal adjustment or equilibration is deemed necessary for other clinical reasons, it should always be planned on articulated study models mounted on a semi-adjustable articulator (Figure 8.1) before irreversible and permanent changes are made to the patient's natural dentition.

In this way, the sequence of alterations can be carefully planned, and it can also be determined whether the desired result is realistically achievable.

It is acknowledged that occlusal treatment can be used successfully to correct an uncomfortable occlusion in a patient with or without TMD. For example, a patient who reports an uncomfortably high, recently placed restoration can be treated with occlusal adjustment of this restoration as the primary treatment.

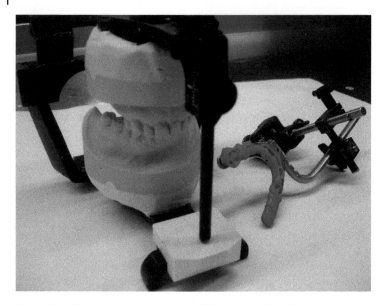

Figure 8.1 Occlusal adjustment or equilibration should always be planned on articulated study models mounted on a semi-adjustable articulator.

Given that there are other, less invasive approaches available and TMD symptoms may be self-limiting, it would seem correct that occlusal adjustment is not indicated unless additional evidence is forthcoming.

Further Reading

Al-Ani, Z. (2020). Occlusion and temporomandibular disorders: a long-standing controversy in dentistry. *Prim. Dent. J.* 9: 43–48.

A l-Ani, Z., Gray, R.J., Davies, S.J. et al. (2005). Stabilization splint therapy for the treatment of temporomandibular myofascial pain: a systematic review. *J. Dent. Educ.* 69 (11): 1242–1250.

Al-Ani, Z., Davies, S., Sloan, P., and Gray, R. (2008). Change in the number of occlusal contacts following splint therapy in patients with a temporomandibular disorder (TMD). *Eur. J. Prosthodont. Restor Dent.* 16 (3): 98–103.

Ash, M.M. and Ramfjord, S.P. (1995). *Occlusion*, 4e. Philadelphia, PA: WB Saunders.

Bales, J. and Epstein, J. (1994). The role of malocclusion and orthodontics in temporomandibular disorders. *J. Can. Dent. Assoc.* 60 (10): 899–905.

Conti, P.C., Ferreira, P.M., Pegoraro, L.F. et al. (1996). A cross-sectional study of prevalence and etiology of signs and symptoms of temporomandibular disorders in high school and university students. *J. Orofac. Pain* 10 (3): 254–262.

De Boever, J.A., Carlsson, G.E., and Klineberg, L.J. (2000). Need for occlusal therapy and prosthodontic treatment in the management of temporomandibular disorders. Part I. Occlusal interferences and occlusal adjustment. *J. Oral Rehabil.* 27 (5): 376–379.

De Boever, J.A., Carlsson, G.E., and Klineberg, L.J. (2000). Need for occlusal therapy and prosthodontic treatment in the management of temporomandibular disorders. Part II: tooth loss and prosthodontic treatment. *J. Oral Rehabil.* 27 (8): 647–659.

Egermark-Eriksson, I., Carlsson, G.E., Magnusson, T., and Thilander, B. (1990). A longitudinal study on malocclusion in relation to signs and symptoms of cranio-mandibular disorders in children and adolescents. *Eur. J. Orthod.* 12 (4): 399–407.

Fricton, J. (2006). Current evidence providing clarity in management of temporomandibular disorders: summary of a systematic review of randomized clinical trials for intra-oral appliances and occlusal therapies. *J. Evid. Based Dent. Pract.* 6 (1): 48–52.

Gray, R. and Al-Ani, Z. (2010). Risk management in clinical practice. Part 8. Temporomandibular disorders. *Br. Dent. J.* 209 (9): 433–449.

Gray, R.J. and Al-Ani, Z. (2013). Conservative temporomandibular disorder management: what do I do? Frequently asked questions. *Dent. Update* 40 (9): 745–756.

Huber, M.A. and Hall, E.H. (1990). A comparison of the signs of temporomandibular joint dysfunction and occlusal discrepancies in a symptom-free population of men and women. *Oral Surg. Oral Med. Oral Pathol.* 70 (2): 180–183.

Kerstein, R. (1996). Occlusion's role in TMD problems? An interview with Dr. Robert Kerstein. *Dent. Today* 15 (3): 68–71.

Klineberg, I. and Jagger, R. (2004). *Occlusion and Clinical Practice: An Evidence-Based Approach*. London: Wright.

Lipp, M.J. (1991). Temporomandibular symptoms and occlusion: a review of the literature and the concept. *J. Colo. Dent. Assoc.* 69 (3): 18–22.

Manfredini, D., Bucci, M.B., Montagna, F., and Guarda-Nardini, L. (2011). Temporomandibular disorders assessment: medicolegal considerations in the evidence-based era. *J. Oral Rehabil.* 38 (2): 101–119.

Manfredini, D., Lombardo, L., and Siciliani, G. (2017). Temporomandibular disorders and dental occlusion. A systematic review of association studies: end of an era? *J. Oral Rehabil.* 44 (11): 908–923.

McNeill, C. (1997). *Science and Practice of Occlusion*. Hong Kong: Quintessence Publishing.

Mohlin, B., Axelsson, S., Paulin, G. et al. (2007). TMD in relation to malocclusion and orthodontic treatment. *Angle Orthod.* 77 (3): 542–548.

Okeson, J.P. (2012). *Management of Temporomandibular Disorders and Occlusion*, 7e. St Louis, MO: Mosby.

Pullinger, A.G., Seligman, D.A., and Gornbein, J.A. (1993). A multiple logistic regression analysis of the risk and relative odds of temporomandibular disorders as a function of common occlusal features. *J. Dent. Res.* 72 (6): 968–979.

Pullinger, A.G. and Seligman, D.A. (2000). Quantification and validation of predictive values of occlusal variables in temporomandibular disorders using a multifactorial analysis. *J. Prosthet. Dent.* 83 (1): 66–75.

Simmons, M. (1997). The validity and utility of disease detection methods and occlusal therapy for temporomandibular disorders. *Oral Surg. Oral Med. Oral Pathol. Oral Radiol. Endod.* 83 (1): 101–106.

Tsukiyama, Y., Baba, K., and Clark, G.T. (2001). An evidence-based assessment of occlusal adjustment as a treatment for temporomandibular disorders. *J. Prosthet. Dent.* 86 (1): 57–66.

Weyant, R.J. (2006). Questional benefit from occlusal adjustment for TMD disorders. *J. Evid. Based Dent. Pract.* 6 (2): 167–168.

Yatani, H., Hatanaka, K., Matsuka, Y. et al. (2002). Multivariate analysis of risk factors in relation to TMD symptoms. *J. Oral Rehabil.* 29 (9): 883.

9

How Would I Adjust a High Occlusal Contact?

Scenario

The patient had a crown fitted recently but has now presented with pain and the tooth is sensitive and tender (Figure 9.1).

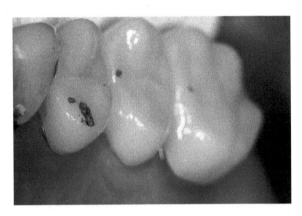

Figure 9.1 This patient had a crown fitted recently but has now presented with pain and the tooth is sensitive and tender.

Rationale

There are several steps to understand before adjusting the restoration or the tooth, and some of these have already been addressed in other chapters:

- Occlusal morphology – Chapter 4.
- Equipment – Chapters 3 and 4.
- Static and dynamic assessment before treatment – Chapter 4.
- Causes and types of high (supraoccluded) occlusal contacts – Chapter 5.

We will discuss in this chapter how to adjust the occlusal contact and the protocols required to remove the right amount so as to not infraocclude the restoration. As master clinicians, we should ensure we have the right equipment and we must also know how to use it and understand its limitations. The objective of adjusting a high spot is to bring the remaining teeth into occlusion and distribute the number of occlusal contacts over as many teeth as possible to share the forces and keep them equal.

Equipment

- Burs.
- Articulating paper and Miller's forceps – covered in Chapters 3 and 4.
- Polishing kit.

Burs

Burs have codes which aid ordering and provide information about the bur.

Shank

- High speed generally uses friction grip shank – code FG.
- Slow speed generally uses right angle latch type shank – code RA.
- Straight handpieces use hand part long straight shank – code HP.

Material

Diamond and tungsten carbide (TC) are the two most common materials in use. Diamonds are measured by grit size and TC use cutting flutes which vary in number. Each has advantages and disadvantages but if used correctly both are effective. In this book we will focus on diamond burs because they are used to adjust enamel, composite, ceramic materials and metal-based restorations whereas TC are mainly used to adjust enamel, composite and metal-based restorations. This varies among companies and a colour-coded system relates to grit size. Table 9.1 shows examples with optimal speed usage for burs.

Table 9.1   Optimal speed usage for burs.

Colour	Grain	Grit size (μm)	Optimal speed (rpm)
White	Ultra fine	8	20 000
Yellow	Extra fine	25	20 000
Red	Fine	46	20 000
Blue	Medium	105–120	160 000
Green	Coarse	126–150	160–300 000
Black	Extra coarse	180–200	160–300 000

The speed usage is crucial because the higher the speed, the greater the removal of material and degradation of the bur. Therefore using 20 μm articulating paper but a green coarse diamond at the required speed means far more removal than the 20 μm paper is measuring. Therefore, the rule is – *same thickness articulating paper as grit size diamond.*

The other factor which requires caution is pressure application so gentle strokes will remove small amounts (precision) and increase the longevity of the bur.

Bur Type

Ideally, we require a bur that can replicate the shape of the tooth that is involved in function (Figure 9.2). The surfaces involved in function are:

- palatal surface of maxillary incisors/canines and incisal edges of incisors
- cusp tips
- cuspal inclines
- marginal ridge.

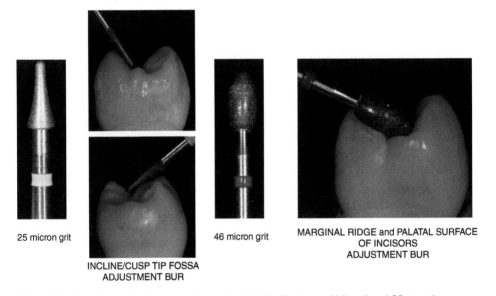

25 micron grit

INCLINE/CUSP TIP FOSSA
ADJUSTMENT BUR

46 micron grit

MARGINAL RIDGE and PALATAL SURFACE
OF INCISORS
ADJUSTMENT BUR

Figure 9.2   Bur shape allowing correct morphological adjustment. Yellow band 25 μm grit.

Articulating Paper

This comes in varying thicknesses. We recommend 20 or 40 μm for restorative work. The rationale is based on precision and minimal invasiveness. When adjusting, our aim is to remove the right spot and right amount.

Polishing Kits

Polishing is an important step to prevent further wear post restoration completion. Different materials have varying finishing protocols and the risk for further damage against the opposing enamel is greater and therefore occlusal instability will occur over time due to the differing wear rates.

- *Non-silica ceramics such as zirconia* – Mitova et al. (2012) have shown that polishing the zirconia post adjustment with diamonds reduces the wear rate on opposing enamel.
- *Silica ceramics such as Empress®, E-max* – Olivera et al. (2006) have also shown that polished ceramics produce less enamel wear.
- *Composite* – this material is weaker than enamel so the objective is to achieve the same surface roughness as enamel. Bansal et al. (2019) have shown that this can be achieved with the polishing systems and involving the marginal enamel is important.

Procedure

How Do We Use This Equipment?

Types of Proud Occlusal Contacts
This classification system is based upon amount of contact area (surface area) of contact and location (Figure 9.3).

Amount of Contact Area
This requires different adjustment processes and is also determined by the thickness of your articulating paper (thinner is better). This also depends upon the existing level of

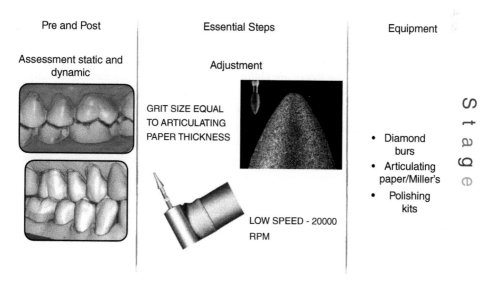

Figure 9.3 Summary of essential steps when adjusting.

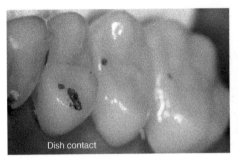
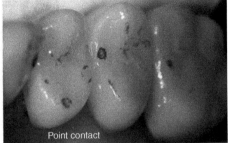

Dish contact

Point contact

Figure 9.4 Dish contact and point contact on an indirect restoration.

tooth wear; if the teeth are flat then you will have a greater contact area, and this is repli-cated in the restoration.

- Point contact – small contact area.
- Dish contact – large contact area (Figure 9.4).

Location

This requires the use of different burs. The location of the proud contact may be on a cusp tip and be a dish contact, for example.

- Fossa.
- Marginal ridge.
- Cuspal incline.
- Cusp tip.
  The location of the static contacts ideally needs to be placed on the:
- fossa, marginal ridge or cusp tip because the forces are axial (through the long axis) avoiding jiggling forces and also restorative materials have great compressive strength but poor tensile strength, *or*
- the restorative material or tooth, *but **not** on*
- cuspal inclines – because the forces are oblique and can cause jiggling forces (mobility) and fracture teeth or restorations
- margins between a restoration and tooth – the material in this area is fragile and thin and therefore prone to rapid deterioration and microleakage.
  So, what is our goal when conforming to the patient's existing occlusion?
- To provide equal contacts on as many teeth as possible in static (i.e. distribute the forces so as to not cause failure of the restoration or other teeth) – swallowing position.
- To provide guidance on cuspal inclines when in dynamic – chewing position.
- To avoid introducing new contacts (unless in a controlled manner) which may strain the adaptive capacity of the patient (Figure 9.5).

The adjustments must be done in supine and seating position because:

- day time – physiological function and parafunction, therefore seated position
- night time – parafunction, therefore supine position.

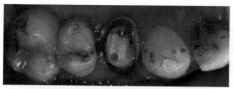

Single crown lost upper right 1st premolar
Static pre assessment - contacts on adjacent teeth

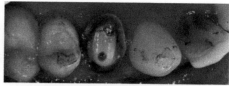

Single crown lost upper right 1st premolar
Dynamic pre assessment - group function

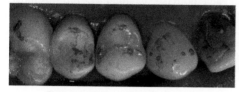

Single crown lost upper right 1st premolar
Static post assessment - contacts on adjacent teeth

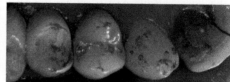

Single crown lost upper right 1st premolar
Dynamic post assessment - group function

Figure 9.5   Restoration of first premolar using occlusal principles.

What is the Outcome of Introducing a New Contact?

Depending upon the adaptative capacity of the individual, this may:

- stimulate a parafunctional habit – system wants to REMOVE
- create new functional chewing movements – system wants to AVOID
- restrict the existing chewing movements – system wants to ACCEPT.

The last option may result in no feedback from the patient, meaning they may not attend for any further treatment and if you review the patient, they may tell you everything is fine.

Principles of Adjustment

It is vital to follow the contours of the tooth – the rationale being that we are simply infraoccluding that high spot but in the right shape corresponding to tooth morphology (Figure 9.6).

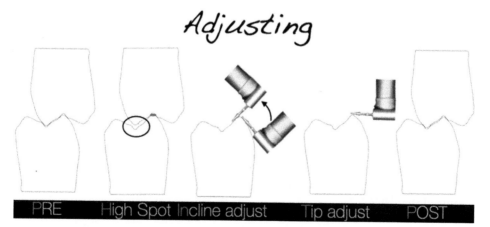

Figure 9.6   How to adjust a high spot maintaining correct morphology.

- For a *proud contact*, whether in static or dynamic, the STOP process must be followed to understand that the postocclusal contacts are different from the preocclusal position. If the proud contact is a point contact then this is removed carefully and the process of asking the patient to tap their teeth together with coloured articulating paper between their teeth is repeated until the contacts on the adjacent teeth are the same as before but the new restoration is incorporated within the system with an occlusal contact. The number of contacts ideally is two – supporting cusp of each tooth (see Chapter 4) – but this must be assessed on a case-by-case basis.
- *Preassessment* includes the following steps.
  - Dry the teeth.
  - Static assessment – dry teeth and tap together with blue (can be any colour) articulating paper held with Miller's forceps.
  - Dynamic assessment – dry the teeth and slide with red (can be any colour but must be different from static) articulating paper held with Miller's forceps either from inside–out or outside–in.
  - Shimstock analysis – shimstock foil held by Miller's forceps is placed on the tooth being restored and the patient is asked to bite together and remain closed. Gently attempt to pull the foil out. If the foil stretches and cannot be pulled out without tearing, then we have a holding contact (meaning the teeth touch). This is repeated with the adjacent teeth and the same tooth on the contralateral side (or a tooth on the opposite side that is contacting).

- The tooth is restored.
- *Postassessment* includes the following steps.

  - Shimstock analysis – shimstock foil held by Miller's forceps is placed on the tooth being restored and the patient is asked to bite together and remain closed. Gently attempt to pull the foil out. If the foil stretches and cannot be pulled out without tearing, then we have a holding contact (meaning the teeth touch). This is repeated with the adjacent teeth and the same tooth on the contralateral side (or a tooth on the opposite side that is contacting). If the restoration is proud then the restored tooth will hold but the adjacent and contralateral teeth will allow the foil to be pulled through. Now we need to mark the point that is proud and this is done using articulating paper.
  - Static assessment – dry the teeth and tap together with blue or black (can be any colour) articulating paper held with Miller's forceps.
  - Dynamic assessment – dry the teeth and slide with red or green (can be any colour but must be different from static) articulating paper held with Miller's forceps either from inside–out or outside–in.

Then adjust – the process for static and dynamic contacts is exactly the same. The key is ensuring you have not introduced a contact that interferes with the static and dynamic movements. For static contact adjustment see Figure 9.7; for incline or dynamic contact adjustment see Figure 9.8.

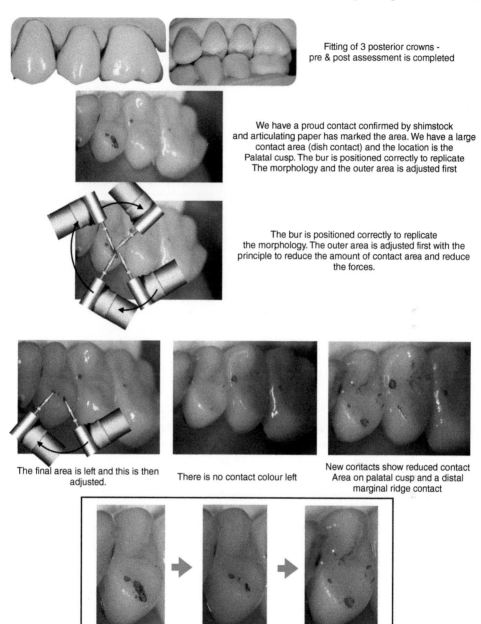

Fitting of 3 posterior crowns -
pre & post assessment is completed

We have a proud contact confirmed by shimstock
and articulating paper has marked the area. We have a large
contact area (dish contact) and the location is the
Palatal cusp. The bur is positioned correctly to replicate
The morphology and the outer area is adjusted first

The bur is positioned correctly to replicate
the morphology. The outer area is adjusted first with the
principle to reduce the amount of contact area and reduce
the forces.

The final area is left and this is then
adjusted.

There is no contact colour left

New contacts show reduced contact
Area on palatal cusp and a distal
marginal ridge contact

Figure 9.7   Clinical case detailing steps on how to adjust a high spot.

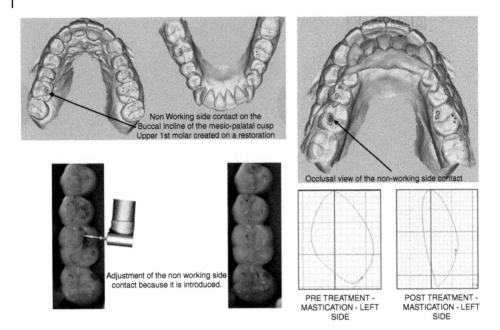

Figure 9.8 Clinical case detailing steps on how to adjust a high spot on a non-working side contact introduced on a bridge.

References

Bansal, K., Gupta, S., Nikhil, V. et al. (2019). Effect of different finishing and polishing systems on the surface roughness of resin composite and enamel: an *in vitro* profilometric and scanning electron microscopy study. *Int. J. Appl. Basic Med. Res.* 9 (3): 154–158.

Mitova, G., Heintzeb, D.S., Walzc, S. et al. (2012). Wear behavior of dental Y-TZP ceramic against natural enamel after different finishing procedures. *Dent. Mater.* 28: 909–918.

Olivera, A.B., Belsuzarri, A., Edmir, M., and Márcia, M.M. (2006). The effect of glazed and polished ceramics on human enamel wear. *Int. J. Prosthodont.* 19 (6): 547–548.

10

How Would I Ensure a Good Occlusion on Posterior Composite Restorations?

You are about to start a cavity preparation for restoring a posterior tooth using composite restoration. What are the principles of good occlusal practice which you would adopt during this operative procedure?

Static Occlusion

The aim is to achieve a stable occlusion on a posterior restoration either when conforming or when reorganising the occlusion. The occlusal contacts on the posterior restoration should provide an intercuspal position (ICP) which is stable and reproducible. This can be achieved when a cusp fits into a fossa or when meeting a marginal ridge which will provide the tooth with axial loading during function.

Premature contacts on cusp inclines should be eliminated as these contacts tend to produce lateral forces on teeth that create undesirable lateral pressure and tension on periodontal tissues. Furthermore, a contact formed against a single cusp slopes, potentially allowing unwanted tilting and overeruption, resulting in an interference in the lateral movement (Figure 10.1).

Axial loading can also be accomplished by tripodization which will offer reciprocal incline contacts. This will create occlusal stability both buccolingually and mesiodistally (Figure 10.2).

When restoring posterior teeth with composite, three discrete contacts around the cusp tip can be achieved for a perfect stable tripodization. This pattern, however, is a time-consuming one and relatively difficult to achieve and in most cases will be lost with time due to restoration wear (Figure 10.3).

The occlusal contacts of a posterior tooth should be marked using thin articulating paper before commencing the cavity preparation (Figure 10.4). This procedure will make it easy to conform to the pre-existing occlusion and will give the operator an idea about the location of the centric stops. It is advisable to avoid involving these centric stops in the cavity preparation whenever possible!

Occlusal contacts occurring at the tooth–restoration interface are undesirable and the opposing occlusal contact should be moved, not removed, to avoid marginal failure (Figures 10.5 and 10.6). The restoration therefore should be planned in such a way that occlusal contact areas are on sound tooth tissue.

Practical Procedures in Dental Occlusion, First Edition. Ziad Al-Ani and Riaz Yar.
© 2022 John Wiley & Sons Ltd. Published 2022 by John Wiley & Sons Ltd.
Companion website: www.wiley.com/go/al-ani-and-riaz/dental-occlusion

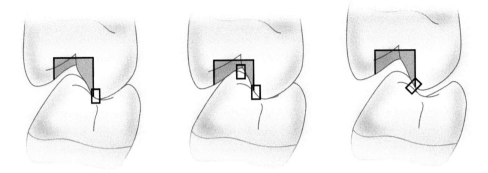

Figure 10.1   A contact formed against a single cusp slopes, potentially allowing unwanted tilting and overeruption, resulting in an interference in the lateral movement.

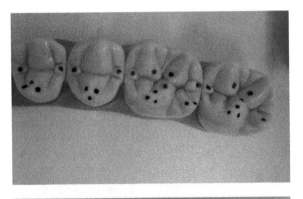

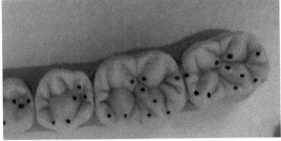

Figure 10.2   Tripodization.

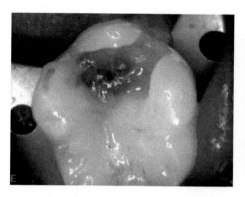
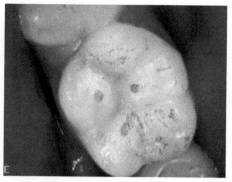

Figure 10.3 Tripodization on a posterior tooth newly restored with composite.

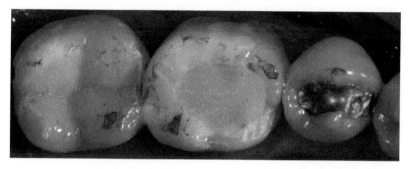

Figure 10.4 The occlusal contacts of a posterior tooth should be marked using thin articulating paper before commencing the cavity preparation.

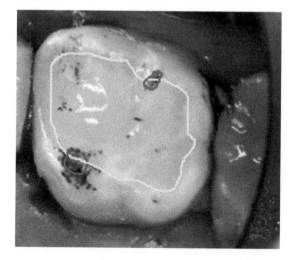

Figure 10.5 Occlusal contacts occurring at the tooth–restoration interface should be avoided.

(a)

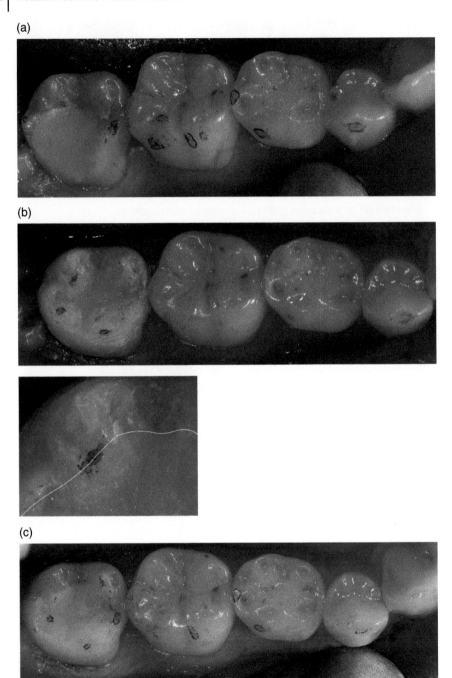

(b)

(c)

Figure 10.6 (a) The best approach is to mark the occlusal contacts of the pre-existing static occlusion before starting the cavity preparation. (b) After tooth preparation and restoring the tooth with composite, the occlusal contacts are checked again, making sure that no new contacts are placed on the tooth–restoration interface. (c) If any occlusal contacts appear to be undesirable, they should be adjusted, and the initial pre-existing occlusal contacts should be reproduced.

Occlusal Surface Morphology and Anterior Guidance

The morphology of the occlusal surfaces of restored posterior teeth is influenced by anterior guidance.

All chewing surfaces should provide 'departure clearance spaces' for the opposing cusps (disclusion during excursive movements) and the practitioner should be familiar with the pattern in which the posterior teeth move across each other in lateral movements. This will facilitate placing the anatomical features of the occlusal surfaces of these teeth in a way which avoids interference during excursions.

When the midbuccal cusp of the lower right first molar moves over the occlusal surface of the upper molar, a crow's foot pattern can be produced on protrusion, working side and non-working side (NWS) movements.

In protrusion, the upper cusp moves distally across the lower molar. In the working side (WS), the upper cusp escapes between the mesiolingual and distolingual cusps of the lower molar. In the NWS excursion, the upper cusp escapes between the mesiobuccal and distobuccal cusps of the lower molar. This is known as the 'crow's foot pattern' (Figure 10.7).

Successive cusp build-up will reduce finishing time and ensure good occlusion by careful attention to progressive reconstruction of natural morphology. You can determine the

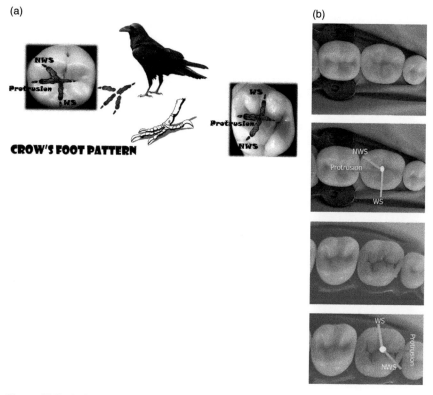

Figure 10.7 (a, b) The crow's foot pattern.

position and depth of fossae, height and position of cusp tips, height, position and morphology of marginal ridges. Landmarks on the adjacent teeth can also give us further small details like wear facets, staining, etc.

Further Reading

Davies, S. and Gray, R. (2002). *A Clinical Guide to Occlusion*. London: British Dental Association.

Lynch, C. (2008). *Successful Posterior Composites: Operative Dentistry*. London: Quintessence.

Nohl, F., Steele, J., and Wassell, R. (2002). Crowns and other extra-coronal restorations: aesthetic control. *Br. Dent. J.* 192: 443–450.

Wassell, R., Naru, A., Steele, J., and Nohl, F. (2015). *Applied Occlusion*, 2e. London: Quintessence.

11

My Front Teeth Feel Loose and Are Moving

Occlusal trauma is defined as 'trauma to the periodontium from functional or parafunctional forces causing damage to the attachment apparatus of the periodontium by exceeding its adaptive and reparative capacities'. It may be self-limiting or progressive.

When examining the patient's static occlusion, the freedom in centric occlusion (long centric) should be examined and noted. This means the ability of the mandible to move anteriorly for a short distance in the same horizontal and sagittal plane while maintaining tooth contact.

In other words, lack of freedom in centric can be detected by placing the finger on the labial surface of the anterior teeth while the patient repeatedly closes and taps the posterior teeth together. Usually, tremors on the upper incisor teeth can be felt when no freedom in centric exists (Figure 11.1).

Occlusal trauma may result from anterior restorations placed on teeth which have no freedom in centric. Palatal surfaces which are too thick will not allow freedom in centric and sometimes patients describe it as 'locked occlusion'. To avoid such a problem, the operator should ensure that the new intercuspal position (ICP) does not incorporate excessively steep cuspal inclines or anterior guidance slope (thick palatal surfaces).

Besides, freedom in centric is an important aspect in implant dentistry where centric platforms in the range of 2–3 mm for posterior opposing supporting cusps must be created. This will minimise the possibility of premature contacts and allow for a more favourable force distribution (Figure 11.2).

Retruded Contact Position Can Be Associated with Occlusal Problems

Fremitus is defined as visible or palpable tooth movements as the teeth come into intercuspal position (ICP) or during mandibular excursion. This can be detected by placing gloved fingers on the upper anterior teeth and asking the patient to tap together (Figure 11.3).

Occasionally, fremitus of the upper incisors can indicate an anterior thrust associated with deflective retruded contact position (RCP)-ICP slide, hence the importance of assessing RCP-ICP slides in patients before commencing any restorative treatment.

Practical Procedures in Dental Occlusion, First Edition. Ziad Al-Ani and Riaz Yar.
© 2022 John Wiley & Sons Ltd. Published 2022 by John Wiley & Sons Ltd.
Companion website: www.wiley.com/go/al-ani-and-riaz/dental-occlusion

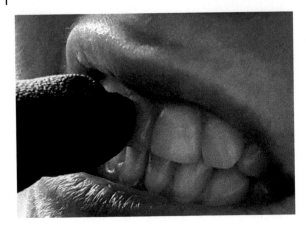

Figure 11.1 Lack of freedom in centric can be detected by placing a finger on the labial surface of the anterior teeth while the patient repeatedly closes and taps the posterior teeth together.

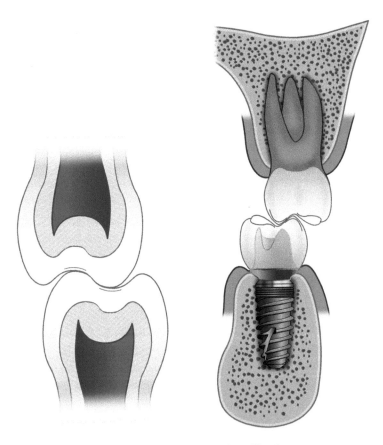

Figure 11.2 'Freedom in centric' natural teeth and implants.

Figure 11.3 Fremitus can be detected by placing gloved fingers on the upper anterior teeth and asking the patient to tap together.

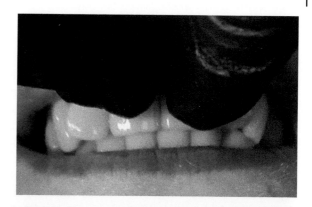

Figure 11.4 Drifting of upper incisors could be a sign of anterior thrust or a deflective RCP-ICP slide.

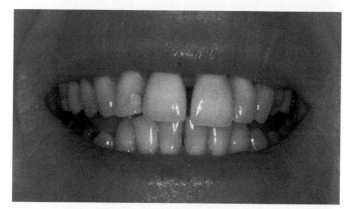

Figure 11.5 Localised palatal wear could be a sign of anterior thrust or a deflective RCP-ICP slide.

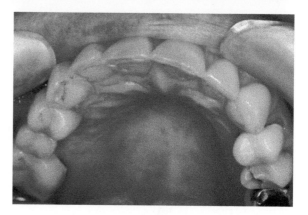

Drifting of upper incisors, localised palatal wear, and damage to restorations could be signs of anterior thrust or a deflective RCP-ICP slide (Figures 11.4 and 11.5).

Generally, if occlusal adjustment of RCP-ICP slide is deemed necessary, it should always be planned on articulated study models mounted on a semi-adjustable articulator before such irreversible and permanent changes are made to the patient's natural dentition.

In this way, the sequence of alterations can be carefully planned, and it can also be determined whether the desired result is realistically achievable.

Conforming to Existing Guidance When Restoring Anterior Teeth: Copying Anterior Guidance

Sound knowledge of tooth morphology is crucial when restoring teeth. When restoring anterior teeth with full crowns, the morphology of the palatal aspects of these teeth should be carefully restored. Incorrectly shaped palatal aspects of these teeth may result in changing the guiding surfaces and will create interference in the protrusive movements. This might cause these anterior teeth to be overloaded, resulting in signs of occlusal trauma such as tooth mobility, localised wear or fractured restorations.

Ideally, satisfactory guidance should be copied into the definitive restorations especially in patients with class II division two incisal relationship when the horizontal space between the upper and lower anterior teeth is very restricted. This can be achieved by several methods.

The custom-made incisal guide table is a simple method which can be utilised to copy the existing guidance into multiple anterior restorations. In this method, accurate facebow and jaw registration records are used to mount preoperative study models on a semi-adjustable articulator. Unset acrylic will be applied on the articulator's incisal table. In combination with the incisal pin, a jig that replicates precisely the shape of the guidance will be constructed. This jig is used to design the palatal surfaces of the new anterior crowns or bridges. This will conform to the shape of the pre-existing anterior guidance before preparation (Figure 11.6).

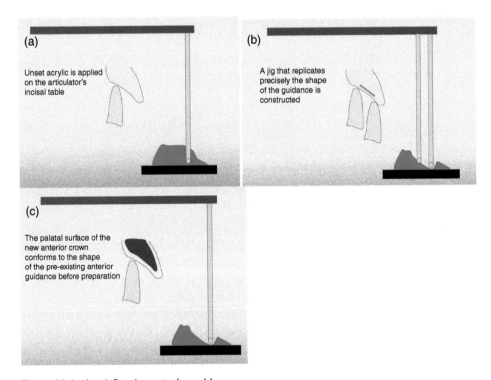

(a)

Unset acrylic is applied on the articulator's incisal table

(b)

A jig that replicates precisely the shape of the guidance is constructed

(c)

The palatal surface of the new anterior crown conforms to the shape of the pre-existing anterior guidance before preparation

Figure 11.6 (a–c) Copying anterior guidance.

Clinical Case

Figure 11.7 shows the procedure of copying the anterior guidance when restoring anterior teeth with a fixed-fixed conventional PFM bridge.

(a)

(b)

(c)

(d)

(e)

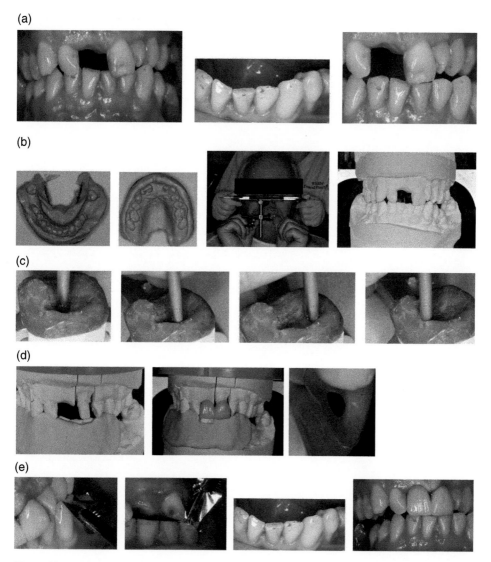

Figure 11.7 (a) Intraoral view of the preoperative case showing marked pre-existing occlusal contacts and protrusive movement. (b) Good impressions, facebow record and mounted casts on a semi-adjustable articlator. (c) A custom incisal guide table is produced guiding the upper model into the same lateral excursions as were present in the teeth before preparation. (d) The models with the prepared teeth are mounted on the articulator and the palatal surfaces of the restorations are shaped in accordance with the movements guided by the custom incisal guide table.
(e) Shimstock is used clinically to check the accuracy of occlusion of the bridge. The occlusal contacts and the protrusive movements are also checked before cementation. The preoperative satisfactory anterior guidance has been successfully copied in the definitive restorations.

Further Reading

Alani, A. and Patel, M. (2014). Clinical issues in occlusion – Part I. *Singapore Dent J.* 35C: 31–38.

Patel, M. and Alani, A. (2015). Clinical issues in occlusion – Part II. *Singapore Dent J.* 36: 2–11.

Wassell, R., Naru, A., Steele, J., and Nohl, F. (2015). *Applied Occlusion*, 2e. London: Quintessence.

12

Canine Guidance or Group Function?

This has been an ongoing debate over many years with discussions on which lateral-based occlusal scheme is the best for the patient. There are four lateral-based occlusal schemes.

- Canine guided occlusion (CGO).
- Group function occlusion (GFO).
- Semigroup function occlusion (sGFO).
- Bilateral balanced occlusion – complete dentures.

Physiologically, you want as many teeth as possible functioning to break the food down and canine guidance is an excursive movement beyond the chewing envelope of function. This chapter will discuss the rationale behind both and how to achieve them clinically.

Ideally, what we want from a lateral-based occlusal scheme is:

- masticatory efficiency – meaning good electromyographic muscle activity, mastication speed and velocity of mandibular movements
- patient comfort and restoration longevity
- reduction of any pathology (parafunction).

The evidence supporting the superiority of one over the other is limited and the study outcomes are based on patient comfort and restoration longevity. Patient comfort is subjective and is based upon the adaptive capacity of the patient. Just because the patient is not experiencing pain doesn't mean we have rehabilitated the patient. The risk is that a reduction in chewing motion occurs which is a guarding mechanism (i.e. a protective role) and therefore the patient has accepted the occlusal scheme but is not performing efficiently, as discussed by Belser and Hannam (1985). Ideally, we aim for a physiologically correct occlusal scheme and provide protection where required when there is pathology (such as parafunction).

The effects on muscle activity are also important because teeth are designed to break food down and the forces required to do so are generated by the muscles. Numerous studies have shown that CGO reduces muscle activity and therefore physiologically we do not want this but when designing a splint to protect our restorations or reduce symptoms from myofascial pain then yes, we want CGO. Abduo and Tennant (2015) concluded that patients successfully adapt to CGO or GFO, but this is the issue – what do we mean by 'successfully adapt?' In the studies, patient acceptance is equated with adaptation and the data are collected using a questionnaire which will be subjective.

Practical Procedures in Dental Occlusion, First Edition. Ziad Al-Ani and Riaz Yar.
© 2022 John Wiley & Sons Ltd. Published 2022 by John Wiley & Sons Ltd.
Companion website: www.wiley.com/go/al-ani-and-riaz/dental-occlusion

A key study by Yi et al. (1996) which discussed the long-term analysis of occlusal factors for more than 10 years was carried out on a cohort of patients who had advanced periodontal disease and were provided with fixed partial dentures. The great majority were satisfied with function – mastication, phonetics, aesthetics, comfort and hygiene – but if your starting point is mobile teeth with missing units then the satisfaction is not linked to occlusal factors alone but rather an improvement from a poor functional starting point.

Canine Guided Occlusion

Introduction

Canine guided occlusion is the vertical and horizontal overlap of the canine teeth which disengages the posterior teeth in excursive movements of the mandible.

It was Dr Angelo d'Amico (1958) who proposed CGO primarily to refute the balanced occlusion theory popular at the time. There is also a debate over whether CGO was discussed by von Spee (1890), though he felt the overbite of the upper canines was an insignificant finding, which lead to Nagao (1919) refuting von Spee's original findings to expand on CGO and to advocate it as he felt bilateral balanced occlusion (BBO) was destructive.

The principle was to look at primate species to prove that CGO was physiologically correct. D'Amico based this upon Dr Gregory's book *Origin and Evolution of the Human Dentition* in which Dr Gregory details the seven stages of evolution of the dentition but for the majority of the stages there are no fossil remains that substantiate the stages. Further analysis by Dr Hector Jones looked at attrition in Pre-white and recent Australian aborigines and he stated that attrition and loss of the canines resulted in an edge-to-edge occlusion. So by providing a class 1 canine relationship which is interlocked between the lower canine and first premolar (still with freedom), we are providing CGO which may protect from wear and this may be true in some individuals who respond by reducing the muscle activity but wear is either physiological or pathological and if caused by parafunction (i.e pathological), giving CGO may not stop that habit. What is interesting is that Dr Jones does discuss group function as the mode of mastication and recognises that in apes, the motion is vertical caused primarily by the large canine so there is an acceptance that CGO will lead to a more vertical/narrower functional movement in humans and other species. Dr D'Amico also states that the 'canine root length is definitely for the purpose of limiting lateral excursions or to act as a stress breaker' and the main objective is to reduce or prevent failure of the restoration and periodontium. If that was the case, then we would simply never see canine wear or mobility.

The clinical application of CGO was firstly initiated by Stuart and Stallard (1959) who ironically were staunch advocates of BBO. Certainly, the canine is important in mastication but how often do we see impacted maxillary canines? These teeth are the most common impaction after third molars and the frequency in the population differs with demographics; for example, the prevalence in a Japanese population is 0.27% but is up to 2.4% amongst Italians, as discussed by Becker and Chaushu (2015).

So which teeth establish the chewing cycle? We simply need to look at the physiology. The permanent teeth that erupt first are the incisors and first molar and it is rare to see impaction or hypodontia of these teeth. The first molar also erupts unopposed by a deciduous tooth, highlighting the importance in mastication. So why do we consider using CGO?

- Restoratively convenient – because we use an articulator which does not replicate the human temporomandibular joint (TMJ), it is easier to build up the palatal surface of the canine to disclude the remaining posterior tooth.
- To reduce muscle activity in patients suffering with myofascial pain and where a stabilisation splint has helped.
- To disclude the posterior teeth where there is a non-working side contact and there are symptoms of reversible pulpitis or cracked tooth syndrome on the posterior tooth (Figure 12.1).

How To Establish Canine Guidance

Using Direct or Indirect Composite, Also Called Canine Risers (Ramp)

This method is done in situ and the patient is the articulator. The objective is to provide a new palatal surface that does not change the static contact but provides steeper guidance to immediately disclude the posterior teeth. In Figures 12.2 and 12.3 note the new inclination of the arrows.

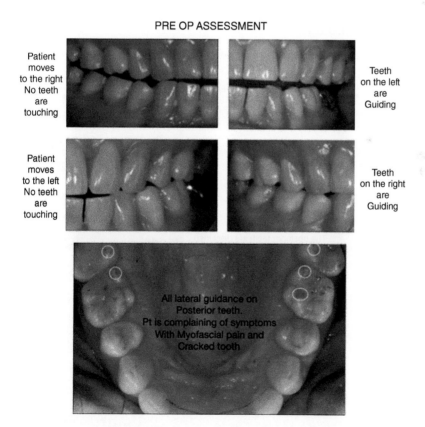

PRE OP ASSESSMENT

Patient moves to the right No teeth are touching

Teeth on the left are Guiding

Patient moves to the left No teeth are touching

Teeth on the right are Guiding

All lateral guidance on Posterior teeth. Pt is complaining of symptoms With Myofascial pain and Cracked tooth

Figure 12.1   Preoperative assessment – all guidance on the posterior teeth.

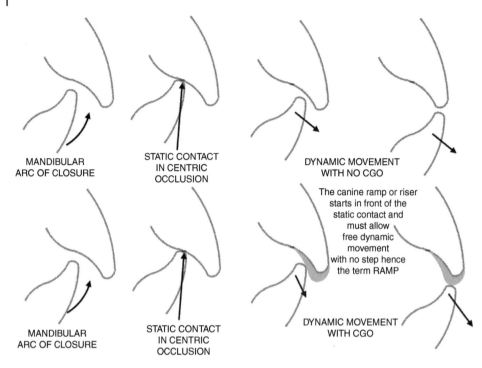

Figure 12.2   Diagrammatic steps detailing how to provide a canine riser.

POST OP ASSESSMENT

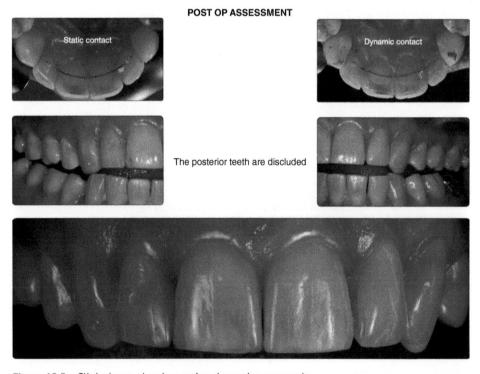

Figure 12.3   Clinical case showing canine riser using composite.

Equipment required is as follows:
- Miller's forceps and articulating paper
- etch/bond/composite.

Using a Laboratory

This will require the use of an articulator which allows for lateral movements so the laboratory will require a facebow record and upper and lower impressions. A bite registration record is generally not needed if the models can be put together by hand easily, otherwise a record will be required. Facebow/articulators and bite registration records are addressed in Chapters 3 and 5.

Equipment required is as follows:

- Miller's forceps and articulating paper
- facebow
- semi-adjustable articulator.

The laboratory provides a functional and aesthetic wax-up. This is transferred to the mouth where any adjustments are completed (Figure 12.4).

What Happens If the Canines are Compromised?

If they are compromised periodontally, structurally or restored with non-retentive restorations or post crowns or bridge pontics, the guidance is best transferred to the premolars or, where possible, create group function between all the teeth in the buccal segment.

Group Function Occlusion

Introduction

Group function occlusion exhibits multiple contacts between maxillary and mandibular teeth in lateral movement on the working side.

The philosophy of group function was advocated by Schuyler (1935) through several of his articles to replace balanced occlusion with unilateral balanced occlusion. Schuyler and other investigators viewed GFO as compensatory adaptation to occlusal wear with the aim of distributing the stresses and thus creating a normal functional relationship. Moses (1952) and Beyron (1954) both suggested that this was 'nature's plan' and therefore beneficial.

How to Establish GFO

Functionally Generated Path Technique (Analogue Method)

This was initially described by Meyer (1959a,b) and has been modified over the years, even as recently as 2018. The principle is to use a coping and place resin on the occlusal surface and ask the patient to make lateral and protrusive movements with the aim of carving the functional pathways from the opposing cusps. The laboratory duplicates this form into the final restoration by creating a custom incisal guidance table (see Chapter 11).

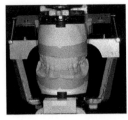

Articulated models - semi adjustable articulator

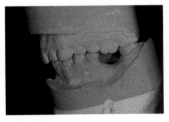

Left lateral view (note over erupted 1st molar)

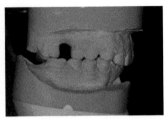

Right lateral view

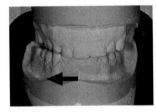

Movement to the right (working side)

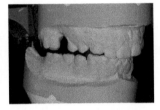

On working side no teeth contact

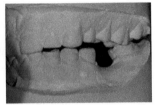

On non working side (left) lower left 2nd molar and upper left 1st molar (over-erupted tooth)

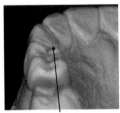

Wax build up of palatal aspect of the canine

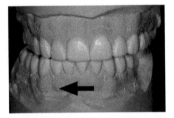

Movement to the right (working side)

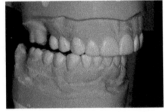

Canines only teeth in contact on working side

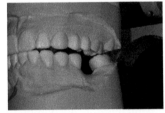

Non working side contact is discluded

Figure 12.4   (a, b) Laboratory stages detailing functional wax-up and canine built up to disclude posterior non-working side contact.

Equipment Required

- Miller's forceps and articulating paper.
- Pattern resin such as DuraLay/brush.
- Facebow.
- Semi-adjustable articulator.

Provisional crowns or a functional mock-up – the same technique as above can be done on provisional crowns using composite and then adjusted.

Stages The steps for this procedure are as follows (Figure 12.5).

1) Laboratory request for resin copings to register functional movements.
2) Remove provisional crowns and try in resin copings. Do not remove all the provisionals in order to maintain occlusal vertical dimension (OVD) and a stable reference point.
3) Apply a drop of liquid resin to the coping to allow for bonding of the new resin with the already set resin. Mix the resin powder with liquid to a thicker consistency and apply while soft to the resin coping.
4) Instruct the patient to bite and start with lateral movements then protrusive.
5) Keep repeating and once the lower cusps have carved the shape, allow to set, remove and disinfect.
6) The laboratory will remount the models using the original mounting and will disengage clasp to allow for movement.
7) Place a resin dough ball into the flat incisal table and start to carve the movements into the resin. This allows waxing up of the new crowns, duplicating the pattern created by the copings and leading to fabrication of definitive restorations.

MODJAW (Digital Method)

No facebow is required for this method (Figures 12.6–12.8).

Making the human fit the mechanical articulator is still a method that many employ today but with the advent of a four-dimensional digital device such as the MODJAW, now we can use the human as the articulator. This device works by placing reflective sensors on the patient, a camera then emits infra-red light and the software calibrates and accurately records the movements of the mandible. These data are recorded and imported into a laboratory design software program such as Exocad. The restorations are then designed and milled from a ceramic block.

Mastication

The movements of mastication are the main reason for the existence of teeth. When we look at CGO and GFO, we generally ask our patients to close together and move their mandible to the working side, be it left or right. This is from a position of closure to open, i.e. inside–out, but our patients do not usually function this way physiologically; rather, they open their mouth and move laterally and close, i.e. outside–in. The movements are split into cycle-in and cycle-out pathways and the incline of cusps is where the contacts are for guidance and breaking the food down.

The process starts with food selection and the incisors capture the food and bring it into the oral cavity, providing a range of information regarding texture, hardness, etc. The food is then transported posteriorly to start the mastication proper. Once the food consistency is thin enough to swallow, indicated by the teeth starting to contact, i.e. periodontal proprioception, the bolus is positioned posteriorly and deglutition proper occurs, transporting the food into the oral pharynx (Figure 12.9).

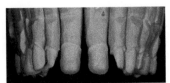
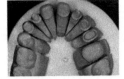
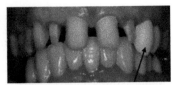

Resin copings made on the prepared model

Resin copings in situ and notes provisional crowns Kept in place to maintain OVD and Centric occlusion

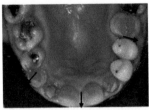
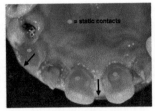
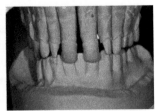

Pattern resin applied and static contacts provided Then patient instructed to make movements

Static contacts with Protrusive and lateral movements

Transferred to laboratory models

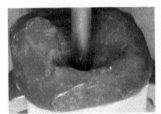
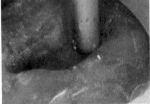
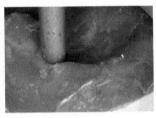

Resin material applied to biting platform table

While the resin is still malleable left lateral movement

Right lateral movement

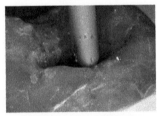

Protrusive movement

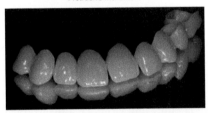

Definitive ceramic restorations

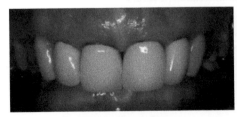
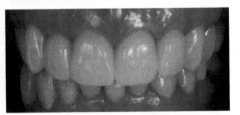

Preoperative Frontal picture

Postoperative Frontal picture

Figure 12.5 Functionally generated pathway technique.

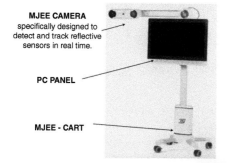

MJEE CAMERA
specifically designed to
detect and track reflective
sensors in real time.

PC PANEL

MJEE - CART

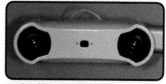

Principle of operation of the camera M-JEE CAM
Here is a simple description of how the camera works:
1. The camera emits infrared light (IR)
2. Infrared light is reflected by reflective markers
3. The camera detects reflected (or emitted) infrared light and transmits the information to the host computer with status information
4. The computer, equipped with the software, extracts the position of each detected point, calculates the 3D position of each detected source, then attempts to match the geometries of known markers.

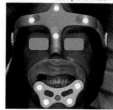

Figure 12.6   MODJAW 4D equipment.

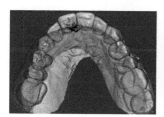 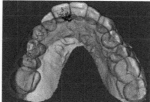 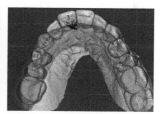

GROUP FUNCTION - designed on exocad

Figure 12.7   Data incorporated within Exocad laboratory software to design restorations.

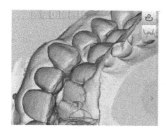 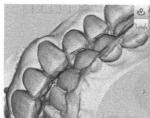 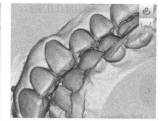

GROUP FUNCTION - assessed after
cementation

Figure 12.8   Group function assessed on MODJAW.

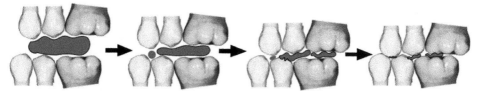

MASTICATION PROPER - THE FOOD IS BROKEN DOWN THROUGH THE MOVEMENTS FROM A THICKER CONSISTENCY TO A THINNER
CONSISTENCY. THE END STAGE OF CHEWING IS WHEN THE TEETH START TO CONTACT SENDING A MESSAGE THAT THE FOOD IS
READY TO SWALLOW

Figure 12.9   Mastication proper.

Masticatory Cycle or The Envelope of Function

From the frontal view, the typical appearance is a pear drop shape (Figure 12.10) but the cycle is controlled by two determinants.

- *Posterior determinants* – this stage of the movement is determined by the TMJ and the muscles of mastication – opening and closing path.
- *Anterior determinants* – this stage is determined by the teeth – cycle in and cycle out.

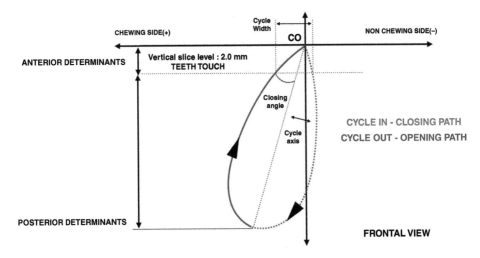

Figure 12.10   Masticatory cycle.

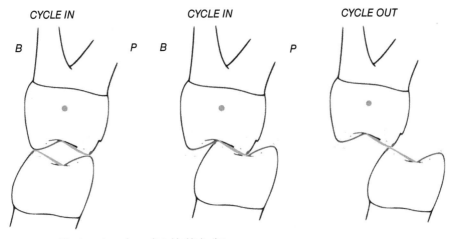

CYCLE IN

B ⎵ P   B ⎵ P

The lower buccal cusp is guided in by the palatal incline of the upper buccal cusp

The upper palatal cusp is guided in by the buccal incline of the lower lingual cusp

CYCLE OUT

The lingual incline of the lower buccal cusp is guided out by the buccal incline of the upper palatal cusp. This is where the crush/shearing of the food occurs and breaks the food down

Figure 12.11   Cycle in–cycle out movements in mastication.

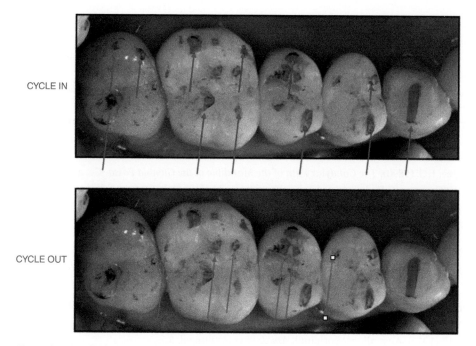

CYCLE IN

CYCLE OUT

Figure 12.12   Clinical case showing replication of masticatory cycle.

Both determinants have an impact on the envelope of function, and this has been shown when providing CGO which narrows this envelope, i.e. the cycle width, also called verticalisation, which includes similar movements seen in other species such as dogs.

When we are designing our restorations, we need to determine where exactly they contact when cycling in and cycling out (Figures 12.11 and 12.12). This is the true goal of rehabilitating the dentition, not just restoring it.

References

Abduo, J. and Tennant, M. (2015). Impact of lateral occlusion schemes: a systematic review. *J. Prosthet. Dent.* 114: 193–204.

Becker, A. and Chaushu, S. (2015). Etiology of maxillary canine impaction: a review. *Am. J. Orthodont. Dentofacial Orthop.* 148 (4): 557–567.

Belser, U.C. and Hannam, A.G. (1985). The influence of altered working-side occlusal guidance on masticatory muscles and related jaw movement. *J. Prosthet. Dent.* 53: 406–413.

Beyron, H. (1954). Occlusal changes in adult dentition. *J. Am. Dent. Assoc.* 48: 674–686.

D'Amico, A. (1958). Canine teeth – normal functional relation of the natural teeth of man. *J. South Calif. Dent. Assoc.* 26: 6–241.

Meyer, F.S. (1959a). The generated path technique in reconstruction dentistry. Part I. Complete dentures. *J. Prosthet. Dent.* 9: 354–366.

Meyer, F.S. (1959b). The generated path technique in reconstruction dentistry. Part II. Fixed partial dentures. *J. Prosthet. Dent.* 9: 432–440.

Moses, C.H. (1952). The significance of stress in the practice of preventive and restorative dentistry. *J. Dent. Med.* 7: 101–103.

Nagao, M. (1919). Comparative studies on the curve of Spee in mammals, with a discussion of its relation to the form of the fosse mandibularis. *J. Dent. Res.* 1: 159–202.

Schuyler, C.H. (1935). Fundamental principles in the correction of occlusal disharmony, natural and artificial. *J. Am. Dent. Assoc.* 22: 1191–1.202.

Stuart, C.E. and Stallard, H. (1959). Diagnosis and treatment of occlusal relations of the teeth. In: *A Syllabus on Oral Rehabilitation and Occlusion* (eds. C.E. Stuart and H. Stallard). San Francisco: University of California.

Von Spee, F.G. (1890). *The Condylar Path of the Mandible in the Glenoid Fossa*. Germany: Kiel.

Yi, S.W., Carlsson, G.E., Ericsson, I., and Wennstrom, J.L. (1996). Long-term follow-up of cross-arch fixed partial dentures in patients with advanced periodontal destruction: evaluation of occlusion and subjective function. *J. Oral Rehabil.* 23: 186–196.

Further Reading

Gregory, W.K. (1922). *Origin and Evolution of the Human Dentition*. Baltimore, MD: Williams & Wilkins.

Jones, H. (1947). Australian Aboriginal. *Am. J. Phys. Anthropol.* 5.

Schuyler, C.H. (1963). The function and importance of incisal guidance in oral rehabilitation. *J. Prosthet. Dent.* 13: 1011–1029.

13

Replacing Missing Teeth – Abutment is Involved with Guidance

Your treatment plan is to prepare upper three and upper five to replace a missing upper premolar with a bridge. The canine has old, failed restorations of amalgam and composite. The upper five is endodontically treated and heavily restored with an amalgam restoration (Figure 13.1).

What are the occlusal considerations which you would adopt before commencing treatment and how is this treatment plan affected by the results of occlusal examination?

The examination of the pre-existing dynamic occlusion revealed that the occlusal scheme in this side is a canine guidance as shown in Figure 13.2. The initial examination will help with the design of the bridge.

Generally, the construction of an indirect restoration requires the accurate transfer of clinically relevant information between the clinician and dental technician. This information, regarding the type and location of the guidance on the canine for example, needs to be reliably transferred to the technician who is going to check it again on the articulator using articulating papers which is the same technique as the clinician uses in the patient's mouth.

Accurate transfer of this information can be done using good-quality photographs or other systems such as sketches or computerised records which have a documented degree of reproducibility.

Different bridge designs can be offered to the patient in this case. The best design, however, is the one conforms to the pre-existing guidance without changing it. There would be no reason to change the occlusal scheme as catastrophic outcomes may result when changing the guidance to an interference. A bulky palatal surface of the canine, in a fixed-fixed bridge design for example, will take the entire masticatory load and may interfere with smooth lateral excursions.

The treatment in this case has been decided to be a fixed-movable bridge design utilising the canine as a mesial abutment with an inlay replacing the two old restorations (minor retainer), and the upper second premolar as a distal abutment (major retainer). The mesial retainer avoids the marked area of canine guidance in dynamic occlusion, allowing the new bridge to conform to this pre-existing guidance without changing it (Figure 13.3).

Practical Procedures in Dental Occlusion, First Edition. Ziad Al-Ani and Riaz Yar.
© 2022 John Wiley & Sons Ltd. Published 2022 by John Wiley & Sons Ltd.
Companion website: www.wiley.com/go/al-ani-and-riaz/dental-occlusion

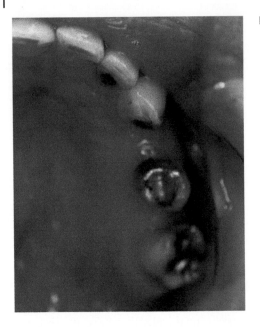

Figure 13.1 Clinical presentation of the case.

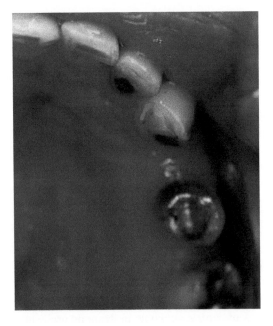

Figure 13.2 Examination of the pre-existing dynamic occlusion revealed that the occlusal scheme in this side is a canine guidance.

A movable non-rigid connector at the mesial end will allow some vertical movement of the mesial abutment tooth. The slight vertical movement of the joint allows the abutment teeth to move independently, a factor that significantly reduces the risk of retainer decementation.

(a)   (b)   (c)

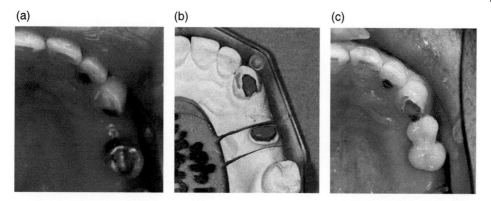

Figure 13.3   (a–c) The design of the restoration can allow the conformative approach to be used in the provision of that restoration.

In addition to conforming to the pre-existing canine guidance in this case, preparations need not be parallel to each other (indicated in tilted abutments).

Generally, if the tooth being restored is involved with guidance and no consideration has been given to conforming to this guidance in the treatment plan, the time needed for occlusal adjustment (chairside) can be excessive.

14

The Space is Lost! Loss of Occlusal Space Following Crown Prep

Your treatment plan is to prepare a last standing upper seven for a full-coverage crown as a retainer to replace a missing upper six and five. During occlusal preparation, an assessment of occlusal space for the restoration is made and it is surprising to see that the preparation is still in contact with its antagonist (Figure 14.1). How has this happened and how can the situation can be rectified?

This situation can be explained by a well-known condition in restorative dentistry called 'the last tooth in the arch syndrome'. The tooth being prepared (upper seven in this example) had previously acted as retruded contact position (RCP) which can be, in many cases, a deflective contact. If the jaw is manipulated to centric relation, the deflective contact will be obvious with the mandible pivoting around it between RCP and intercuspal position (ICP). This contact forms a posterior fulcrum when the patient occludes, initiating a slide from RCP to ICP, and causes the mandible to pivot into the intercuspal position. Normally on closing into the ICP, the patient subconsciously steers around this deflective contact.

When the occlusal surface of the last tooth in the arch is prepared for a crown, the deflective contact (the previous landmark) into ICP will be removed. When closing, the condylar heads are no longer 'guided' by the previous RCP into their 'usual' position in ICP. As this happens, the condyle moves away from its centric relation, taking a more superior position. Ultimately, this will lead to losing the occlusal clearance for the crown (Figure 14.2).

Dealing with This Problem Clinically

Technique 1

After detecting the pivoting contact on the tooth to be crowned, a greater reduction of the occlusal surface of the abutment should be performed. Following preparation, a provisional crown should be fitted in the first visit followed by a final impression and jaw registration in the following visit. The occlusal clearance should then be assessed for the need for more reduction should there be an alteration of jaw position in the interim.

Practical Procedures in Dental Occlusion, First Edition. Ziad Al-Ani and Riaz Yar.
© 2022 John Wiley & Sons Ltd. Published 2022 by John Wiley & Sons Ltd.
Companion website: www.wiley.com/go/al-ani-and-riaz/dental-occlusion

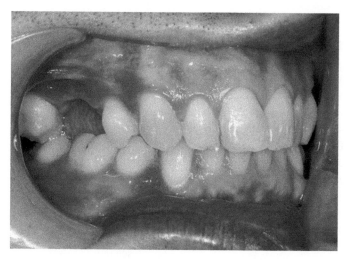

Figure 14.1   Clinical presentation.

(a)

(b)

(c)

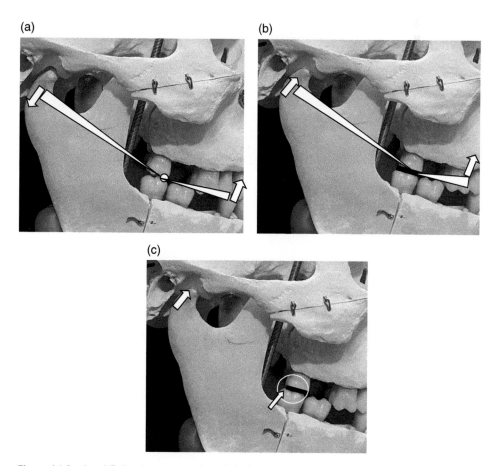

Figure 14.2   (a–c) Following preparation of the last tooth for a crown, the condyle moves away from its centric relation, taking a more superior position which causes loss of occlusal clearance.

Technique 2

Remove RCP contact and defer final impression and jaw registration for 2 weeks.

Technique 3 (Island Technique)

The RCP contact should be marked with an articulating paper and noted (Figure 14.3). When preparing the tooth, this RCP contact should be kept as a pillar protruding from the prepared tooth (Figure 14.4). A definitive impression will be taken as normal.

A provisional crown with a hole in it should be placed using a sectional matrix in the usual way. The RCP contact will appear as an island protruding from this hole. This island will act as an 'occlusal stop' to prevent condylar repositioning (Figure 14.5).

After articulation of the casts and before fabrication of the definitive restoration, the technician should remove this occlusal stop to create the ideal morphology of the occlusal surface of the prepared tooth. In order for the clinician to remove the same amount of the occlusal stop from the prepared abutment clinically, a transfer coping can be useful here.

(a)   (b)

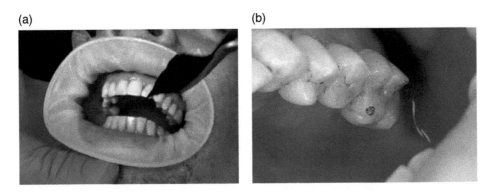

Figure 14.3   (a, b) Marking RCP contact.

(a)   (b)

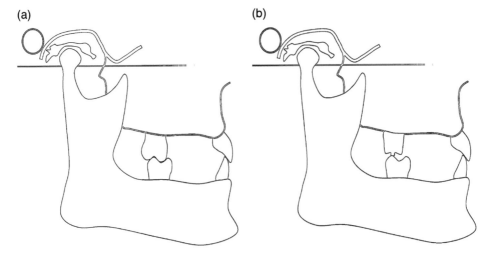

Figure 14.4   (a, b) The island technique.

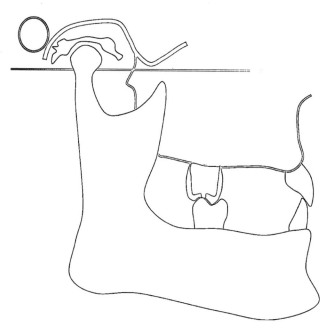

Figure 14.5   The RCP contact appears as an island protruding from the crown to act as an 'occlusal stop' to prevent condylar repositioning.

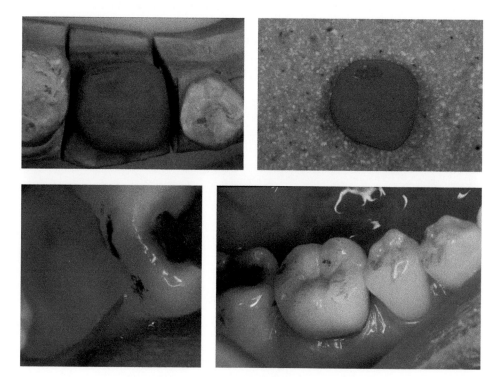

Figure 14.6   The transfer coping in use in the laboratory and clinically.

In the laboratory, a coping made of a rigid-setting material (such as DuraLay) can be placed over the entire tooth surface, and perforated in situ over the island to fit the adjusted height of the preparation.

The coping can now be removed, and the restoration may now be contoured and fabricated as normal.

At the chairside, the temporary restoration should be removed carefully and the same coping used in the laboratory is placed over the tooth. The protruding occlusal stop can now accurately be removed, and the definitive restoration is fitted and cemented on the abutment (Figure 14.6).

Further Reading

Ali, K. and Addison, T. (2019). Managing 'last tooth in the arch syndrome' and restoring retruded contact position. *Dent. Update* 46: 438–449.

Blair, F., Wassell, R., and Steele, J. (2002). Crowns and other extra-coronal restorations: preparations for full veneer crowns. *Br. Dent. J.* 192: 561–571.

Davies, S. and Gray, R. (2002). *A Clinical Guide to Occlusion*. London: British Dental Association.

Nohl, F., Steele, J., and Wassell, R. (2002). Crowns and other extra-coronal restorations: aesthetic control. *Br. Dent. J.* 192: 443–450.

Wassell, R., Naru, A., Steele, J., and Nohl, F. (2015). *Applied Occlusion*, 2e. London: Quintessence.

Wilson, P. and Banerjee, A. (2004). Recording the retruded contact position: a review of clinical techniques. *Br. Dent. J.* 196: 395–402.

15

My Front Teeth are Worn

Scenario

The patient presented with chipped and worn front teeth. They are occasionally sensitive, but the patient is embarrassed to smile and reluctant to bite into anything (Figure 15.1).

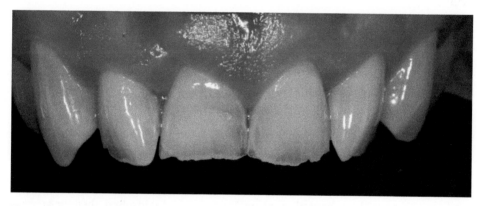

Figure 15.1   Initial presentation.

Rationale

Tooth surface loss (TSL) or tooth wear (TW) is multifactorial with a complex aetiology. The general consensus is that one or more factors contribute. When formulating a diagnosis and treatment plan, the cause and nature of the wear must be considered.

Types of Tooth Surface Loss

There are four types of TSL: abrasion, abfraction, attrition and erosion.

Practical Procedures in Dental Occlusion, First Edition. Ziad Al-Ani and Riaz Yar.
© 2022 John Wiley & Sons Ltd. Published 2022 by John Wiley & Sons Ltd.
Companion website: www.wiley.com/go/al-ani-and-riaz/dental-occlusion

Abrasion

Abrasion is defined by Addy and Shellis (2006) as caused by the sliding or rubbing of abrasive external objects against the tooth surface. Prevalence of 28–62% is seen in the literature. Other factors such as erosion (chemical abrasion) and abfraction may also play a role.

- *Aetiology* – vigorous brushing with an abrasive toothpaste and hard bristles or abrasive foods such as vegetables not washed and therefore containing traces of soil and habits such as nail biting, holding hair pins or thread biting will cause abrasion on the involved tooth surface.
- *Appearance* – clinically seen on multiple teeth as V-shaped notches in the cervical region with smooth surfaces and sharply defined margins often combined with gingival recession.

Abfraction

Grippo et al. (2004) defined afraction as a wedge-shaped or grooved lesion appearing in the cemento-enamel junction (CEJ) and caused by eccentrically applied occlusal forces that lead to dental flexion but it was Lee and Eakle in 1984 who proposed the dental flexion hypothesis.

- *Aetiology* – this is multifactorial involving erosion and occlusal forces. In combination with non-bacterial acids, the term 'stress corrosion or biocorrosion' is used. These lesions appear where there is no gingival recession so abrasion cannot be involved in abfraction aetiology. The lesions can also be seen subgingival, again eliminating toothbrush abrasion. There are predisposing factors such as bone fenestration and dehiscence and the most common teeth to be involved are the canines and premolars which have thin crestal bone as discussed by Cuniberti and Rossi (2019). A recent finite element study by Stănuşi et al. (2020) looking at stress generated in the enamel of the upper first premolar found higher stress in the cervical area mainly on the buccal side which may explain why abfraction is mainly seen on the buccal surface.
- *Appearance* – wedge shaped with sharp margins but localised to a small number of teeth and can be seen with no gingival recession. If erosion is also involved, then the appearance varies but there is no consensus on what that is.

Attrition

Defined by Davies et al. (2002) as the wear process of tooth tissue by direct tooth–tooth contact. Several factors predispose to increase in wear such as coarse porcelain opposing natural teeth or loss of posterior teeth leading to occlusal collapse.

- *Appearance* – well-defined wear facets on the surfaces of teeth in one jaw which match the corresponding facets on opposing teeth in the other jaw when performing eccentric movements.

Erosion

Defined by Pindborg (1970) as a chemical dissolution of hard tissues which is not related to bacterial plaque.

The prevalence of TSL or TW is increasing, with acidic drinks widely considered to be the major factor in children. In 2013, 44% of 15 year olds showed evidence of TSL on the palatal surface of incisors and 31% had TSL on the occlusal surface of first permanent molars. This was an 11% increase from 33% in 2003. The risk is that this may continue into adulthood. On a global level, the prevalence of erosion is between 20% and 45% (most recordings done clinically) with dentine involvement in 2–45% with a general trend that males are affected more.

- *Aetiology* – exogenous or endogenous acids.
  - Endogenous – gastric acid (via vomiting or reflux episodes) known as gastro-oesophageal regurgitation disorder (GORD). It has been reported by Bartlett et al. (1996) that 64% of palatal erosion is related to GORD. of which 30% are silent refluxers. Other signs include heartburn, chronic cough or laryngitis. Predisposing factors include alcohol, pregnancy, obesity and hiatus hernia.
  - Exogenous – special diets, acidic drinks such as wine, carbonated drinks and citrus juice and foods, abuse of drugs and alcohol, occupation exposure to acids and swimming pools with poorly buffered chlorine sterilisation. Some mouthwashes have a pH below 5.5 (critical pH of enamel). Several medications causing reduced salivary flow, such as antidepressants and sedatives, Sjögren's syndrome or head and neck radiotherapy can predispose a patient to dental erosion.

- *Appearance* – described by Carvalho et al. (2016) in the consensus report by the European Federation of Conservative Dentistry.

  - Rounded edges are typically seen.
  - Cupping (concavities) of cusps and flattening of occlusal structures.
  - Lingual and labial smooth surfaces are flattened.
  - An intact rim of enamel along the gingival margin may be present.
  - A reduction in the occlusal vertical dimension (OVD) if no dentoalveolar compensation occurs.
  - A proud restoration such as amalgam.
  - Lesions may affect enamel only or may extend into dentine.
  - Lesions can be localised to a few teeth or generalised with varying symmetrical or asymmetrical distribution (Figure 15.2).

How Does Saliva Play a Role in Tooth Surface Loss?

The main role of saliva is its buffering capacity and there are interindividual variations. There are three buffering systems.

- The bicarbonate system – bicarbonate concentration is dependent upon flow rate.
- The phosphate system – remineralisation.
- The proteins – pellicle layer.

Dentoalveolar Compensation

There are two reactions to TSL.

- Passive tooth eruption with bone remodelling and growth.
- Lack of bone remodelling which may lead to a loss in OVD.

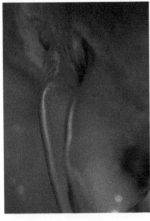
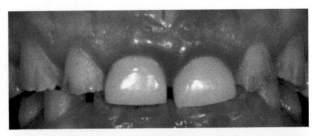
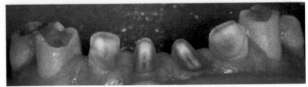

Abrasion caused by a firm
toothbrush - note the grooved
appearance

Attrition primarily caused by parafunction
Note the increased wear when opposed to porcelain

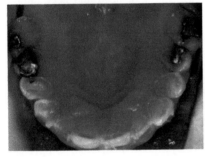
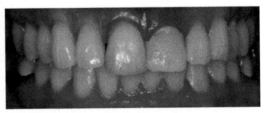

Erosion caused by reflux and note
the surfaces affected are the palatal surfaces

Abfraction lesions on the canines and premolars only.
Note gingival inflammation so unlikely to be abrasion

Figure 15.2   Tooth surface loss and tooth wear.

What is the impact of dentoalveolar compensation?

- *Function* – there is an impact on bite force when OVD is reduced with patients having a significantly lower maximum bite force when compared to patients without attrition as shown by Jain et al. (2013).
- *Aesthetics* – the aesthetic consequences on facial morphology manifest as altered facial contour, narrowed vermillion borders and overclosed commissure with mandibular prognathism.

Crothers and Sandham (1993) reported differences in vertical facial dimensions as a result of severe dental wear. They noted a reduction in lower face height and increase in upper face height and therefore the total face height remained unchanged. This is dentoalveolar compensation (DAC).

We have now lost tooth structure and therefore space to replace it. We must increase the OVD to replace what has been lost. Increasing the OVD will also affect the facial profile with the major changes occurring in the lower face height. This is subjectively judged as a positive change with patients showing an increased happiness with their orofacial appearance post dental rehabilitation involving an increase in OVD.

Constricted Chewing Pattern (CCP)

These patients have no freedom in centric occlusion, i.e. they have a restricted envelope of function also described as a constricted chewing pattern (CCP). What is freedom in centric occlusion? This is when the patient can bite on their posterior teeth in centric occlusion and can slide forwards a small fraction before contacting the anterior teeth. The same is true for lateral movements, also called wide centric. The Glossary of Prosthodontics Terms calls this the intercuspal contact area – the range of tooth contacts in maximal intercuspal position. Patients who parafunction have a greater range of movement and the restorations need to allow this and therefore the cuspal inclinations will be flatter and the fossa shape will be wider.

Patients with a CCP present with chipped/worn anterior teeth and temporomandibular joint (TMJ) symptoms.

Patients who generally do not have freedom in centric:

- are Class 2 div 2
- have received restorative treatment which has resulted in reclining of the incisors or providing bulky cingulums on the anterior indirect restorations
- have had orthodontic treatment which has involved retraction of the anterior teeth normally associated with loss of the premolars.

Test

Ask the patient to sit upright and close together with shimstock foil between the anterior teeth. The shimstock foil cannot be pulled through. Then ask the patient to tilt the head backwards and this should allow the condyle to move posteriorly, making space anteriorly but in a CCP there is no space because the condyle has been pushed distally due to the position of the anterior teeth and they still hold shimstock foil (Figures 15.3 and 15.4).

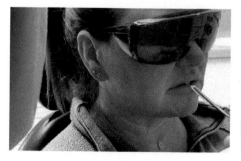
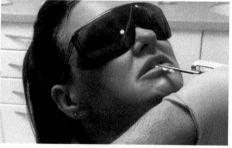

Shimstock hold on anterior
teeth when sitting upright

Head tilted backwards
Shimstock hold on anterior
teeth indicates constricted
chewing

Figure 15.3   CCP test.

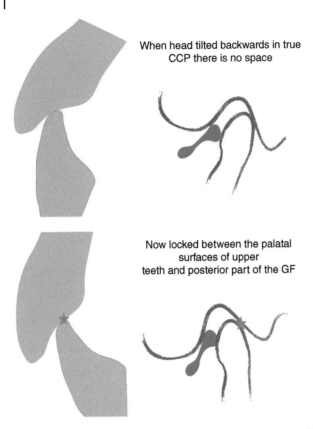

When head tilted backwards in true
CCP there is no space

Now locked between the palatal
surfaces of upper
teeth and posterior part of the GF

Figure 15.4   Diagram showing the condyle against the posterior wall of the glenoid fossa.

Procedure

Management of CCP involves recreating the anterior space (Figure 15.5).

Options

1) Orthodontics to move the upper anterior teeth labially or the lower anterior teeth lingually.
2) If restorative indirect treatment is in situ then adjustment with 200 μm paper while the patient is chewing is done until there are no marks on the palatal aspect of the upper anterior teeth or labial aspect of the lower anterior teeth.

Management of Tooth Surface Loss

The evidence-based literature does not provide strong conclusions when presenting treatment options for TSL or TW as discussed by Muts et al. (2014) in a systematic review.

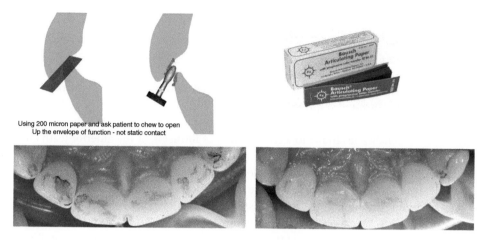

Using 200 micron paper and ask patient to chew to open
Up the envelope of function - not static contact

Figure 15.5 Restorative correction; see option 2 for explanation.

To address management, this chapter will concentrate on localised wear with a specific focus on anterior teeth because the greater degree of wear occurs here (Pigno et al. 2001).

The management is linked to the cause, complexity, amount of wear and whether active or not.

Objectives of Treatment

- Reduce or stop progression of the advanced lesion.
- Reduce symptoms of pain and dentine hypersensitivity.
- Restore aesthetics.
- Restore function.
- Improve quality of life.

Minimal Wear

Dietary changes (if the cause), referral to a medical practitioner if GORD is suspected.

Monitoring using scratch test, study models, digital scans and photographs. Prevention using fluoride exposure, casein–phosphopeptide-stabilised amorphous calcium phosphate (CCP-ACP). Restorative – simple restorations using composite to seal erosion cavities or restore incisal edges.

Moderate and Severe Wear

All of the above with a greater focus on restorative management using direct or indirect composite. With localised tooth wear, our focus is to rebuild the anterior teeth. There are two methods. We can maintain CO by creating the necessary interocclusal space for the restorations by further occlusal reduction; however, this will have severe repercussions for pulpal health, resistance and retention form for the restorations and limits future options. Crown lengthening is an option but requires careful planning and is not without additional complications. Therefore, creating the additional space requires an increase in OVD and a reorganised approach, because we open in an arc and therefore we use centric relation (see Chapter 3 for methods of recording CR) as our reference point because in centric occlusion there is no space.

If we restore the anterior teeth only at an increased OVD, what happens to the posterior teeth because they are out of contact? This is known as the Dahl concept proposed by Dahl et al. (1975). Over a period of time (4–6 months but can take up to 24 months), the posterior occlusion re-establishes itself due to a combination of intrusion of the anterior teeth and eruption of the posterior teeth.

Increasing the OVD also has a favourable biomechanical advantage by reducing the incisal guidance angle which also reduces the off-axial forces (Figure 15.6).

When rebuilding the anterior teeth, we must understand the morphology so that this can be recreated in the restorations. The literature provides us with ideals, and these must be analysed with the facial proportions of the patient, with the smile at rest and when smiling. The perceptions of clinicians and laypersons are different so we must tread carefully when prescribing a smile.

There are some important criteria to bear in mind when assessing and rebuilding of the smile and increasing OVD.

- Facial analysis.
- Healthy TMJ and muscles.
- Aesthetic analysis – dentolabial and dental.
- Functional analysis – occlusal plane, phonetics, anterior guidance.
- Centric relation – see Chapter 3.

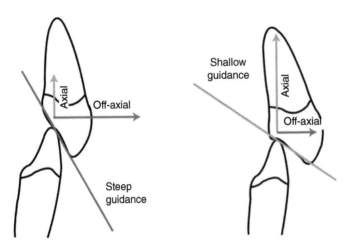

Figure 15.6 Anterior bite platform created using the Dahl concept with the change in incisal guidance and forces. *Source:* Reproduced with permission from Mizrahi B. The Dahl principle: creating space and improving the biomechanical prognosis of anterior crowns. Quintessence Int 2006;37:245–251.

Facial Analysis

Examine	Procedure	Objective
Horizontal reference lines (HRL)	Full face frontal picture	Incisal plane is parallel with HRL
Vertical reference lines (VRL)	Full face frontal picture	Axial inclination of the incisors is coincident with the VRL
Facial proportions	Full face frontal picture	When assessing OVD, has there been DAC?

DAC, dentoalveolar compensation; OVD, occlusal vertical dimension.

The facial analysis allows us to assess features that place the dentition in the correct space in relation to the face. We use horizontal reference lines (HRL) and vertical references lines (VRLs) and facial proportions when looking frontally and from a lateral aspect, the profile, E-line and nasiolabial angle provide us with information at the starting point. The presence of moderate or slight irregularities does not compromise the result as long as certain criteria are met.

Horizontal Reference Lines

- *Horizon* (H) – this is the surface of the earth or the horizontal reference on the articulator.
- *Interpupillary line* (IP) – a horizontal line running between the pupils of the left and right eyes.
- *Commissural line* (CS) – a horizontal line running between the corners of the mouth.

Generally, the interpupillary line is taken as the reference for horizontal but in cases where the eyes or corner of the mouth are not positioned at the same height then the horizon is taken as the ideal plane regardless of alignment with interpupillary and commissural lines, but this cannot be absolute. If the interpupillary and commissural lines are parallel they can be used as a reference for restorative rehabilitation. Therefore, the correct use of the facebow will replicate the clinical situation.

Vertical Reference Lines

The facial midline is the glabella, tip of nose and chin but this is not always reliable so the centre of the upper lip is the ideal reference point for the facial midline (Figure 15.7).

The face is split into three portions or thirds (Figure 15.8).

- Upper third – hairline and ophraic line (eyebrows).
- Middle third – ophraic line to interalar line (nose).
- Lower third – interalar line to the tip of the chin.

The lower third receives the greatest attention when the OVD is reduced. When increasing the OVD, in a short face the profile can be improved but in a long face the appearance could be worsened which is why we look at the facial profile.

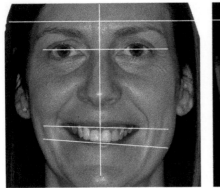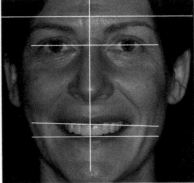

Figure 15.7 Vertical and horizontal reference lines. This photo shows the IP line and CS not being parallel. Note that the occlusal plane is canted. In this rehabilitation we will use the IP plane (also parallel with H). The vertical midline is correct (note that the incisal plane is corrected).

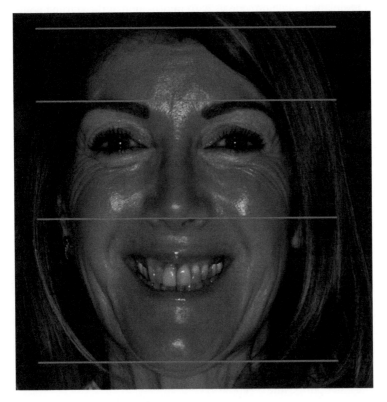

Figure 15.8 Facial proportions.

A healthy TMJ and muscles (Figure 15.9) are crucial before embarking on treatment. There must be no muscle or TMJ pain. Joint loading and sleep apnoea are important tests when restoring the anterior teeth, especially if a CCP is suspected.

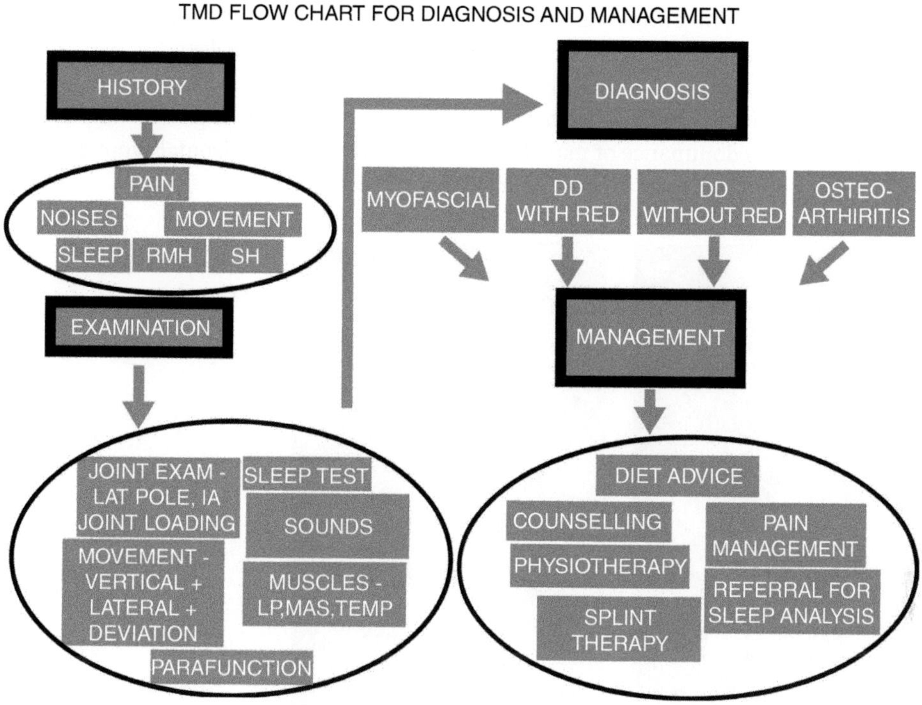

TMD FLOW CHART FOR DIAGNOSIS AND MANAGEMENT

Figure 15.9 Detailed TMD flow chart.

Aesthetic Analysis

Photographs and videos aid this process.

- *Dentolabial aspect* – the lips hide or expose the teeth. We look at the static and dynamic movements of the lip and the exposure of teeth.
- *Lip mobility* – action of the orbicularis oris should be assessed; if too active, this can retract the lip and expose more tooth and gum. Reduced activity (due to embarrassment and training) shows less tooth and gum.
- *Maxillary arch position* – this also has an impact on lip and tooth position. When you have a normal size central but no tooth display at rest and minimal lip mobility, it can be due to a upper lip length being too long. The other thing to consider when you have a normal central and no minimal display is whether the teeth and alveolus may be retruded. The resting position of the lip is highly influenced by the underlying skeletal structures, so if the patient has a maxillary deficiency in terms of anterior projection of the maxilla, the net result will be minimal tooth display and reduced lip mobility. This can also occur if the maxilla is normal but the teeth are retruded, as can sometimes happen following premolar extraction and retraction of the maxillary anteriors.
- *The E-line and nasolabial angle* provide information with regard to lip position (Figure 15.10). The E-line joins the tip of the nose to the tip of the chin. According to Ricketts (2009), the upper lip is 4 mm posterior and the lower lip is about 2 mm but there is significant variation between sexes, races, etc. The nasolabial angle is formed by two

intersecting lines, one on the base of the nose and the other on the outer edge of the upper lip. Normal profiles are 90–95° in males and 100–105° in females.

- The lip volume also has an impact on tooth shape.
  - Average lip volume – anterior teeth well proportioned in terms of shape and dimension.
  - Thin lips – less dominance of maxillary central incisors with horizontal symmetry.
  - Full lips – marked dominance of the maxillary central incisors.

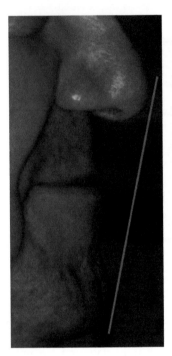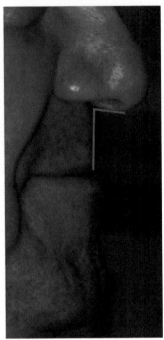

Figure 15.10   E-line and nasio-labial angle.

Dental Analysis

Examine	Procedure	Objective
Tooth exposure at rest	Simply ask the patient to breathe through their mouth and analyse the amount of incisal visibility for both upper and lower central incisors	Assesses incisal visibility using guidelines and provides information with regard to the amount of tooth loss and whether to add material or orthodontically intrude or crown lengthen
Incisal edge	Ask the patient how they would smile 'if they won the lottery'	To establish the correct incisal curvature and aid re-establishment of anterior guidance providing posterior disclusion
Smile line	Ask the patient how they would smile 'if they won the lottery'	Determines incisal visibility and therefore whether to add material to anterior teeth or orthodontically intrude or crown lengthen
Incisor shape, size and proportion for upper and lower central incisors	Periodontal probe or digital callipers are used to measure the width and length	To determine ideal function and aesthetics

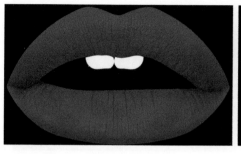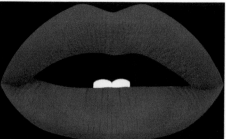

Figure 15.11   Incisal view at rest.

Tooth Exposure at Rest
The following measurements are given as a guide.

- Maxillary central incisors – this varies between 1 and 5 mm but as a guide: males – 2 mm, females – 4 mm. Younger patients show much more than middle-aged patients and this is due to wear and reduction in muscle tone.
- Mandibular central incisors – an ideal value of 1–3 mm. Younger patients show less than middle-aged patients and due to reduction in muscle tone.
- Static – lips at rest (Figure 15.11). Simply ask the patient to breathe through their mouth and analyse the amount of incisal visibility.

Incisal Edge
The incisal plane is generally convex and follows the upper border of the lower lip.

Smile Line
Tjan et al. (1984) identified three types of smile lines.

- Low smile line – exposure of anterior teeth by no more than 75%.
- Average smile line – 75–100% of anterior teeth including interdental papillae.
- High smile line – anterior completely exposed including gingival band of varying height.

A high smile line is found in twice as many female subjects and this is partly due to the length of the upper lip which is generally 2 mm shorter.

Incisor Shape/Size and Proportion
- *Shape* – three shapes – triangular, ovoid and square.
- *Size* – on average:

  - Width – 8.3–9.3 mm.
  - Length – 10.4–11.2 mm.

The width generally remains constant and this provides us with a proportion that can be calculated when wear has occurred.
Proportion – the width of the central incisor is generally 75–80% of the length (Figure 15.12).

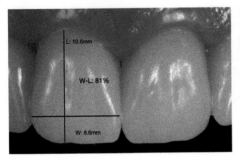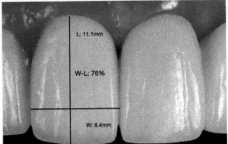

Figure 15.12 Central incisor proportions.

Symmetry between both central incisors is not typical in nature but aesthetics is based upon this principle so we aim to deliver symmetrical incisors.

Functional Analysis

Examine	Procedure	Objective
Occlusal plane/incisal plane	Accurate impressions, facebow record, interocclusal registration in CR and full-face retracted view picture	To develop ideal function and aesthetics by harmonising parallelism between the occlusal plane and the HRL
Phonetics	Video recording articulating words M – Emma E – EEEEEE F – Fifty five S – Sixty six	Provides information regarding visibility and position of the incisal edge in relation to the lips. OVD can also be determined and we do not want to alter patient's speech
Joint loading and sleep apnoea	Tongue spatula or leaf gauge	A healthy joint can take unlimited loading, but an inflamed joint cannot. We want to ascertain health before embarking on restorative treatment
Anterior guidance	Ask patient to move the mandible forward and laterally from either a closed or open position	The skeletal and incisal relationship will determine whether treatment is possible (a Class 3 skeletal patient is more difficult to treat). Overjet and overbite provide necessary data when planning an increase in OVD

CR, centric relation; HRL, horizontal reference line; OVD, occlusal vertical dimension.

Occlusal Plane/Incisal Plane

This is a line running from the central incisors to the canines and the maxillary first molars. The incisal plane is the anterior portion of the occlusal plane and needs to be parallel to the HRLs of the face (Figure 15.13).

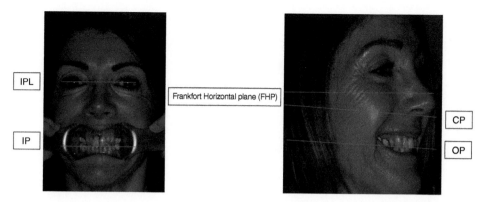

Figure 15.13 (a) Occlusal and incisal plane. A full face frontal retracted view allows analysis of the IP line and incisal plane being parallel. (b) The occlusal plane (OP) is normally parallel to Camper's plane (CP).

Edentulous Patients

The occlusal plane is generally parallel to Camper's plane which is the inferior border of the ala of the nose traced posteriorly to the superior border of the tragus, and this is more important in complete denture fabrication. The correlation between this and Frankfort's plane forms an angle of roughly 10°.

Dentate Patients

Frankfort's Plane (FP)

On a cephalometric analysis, this is a line traced between porion and orbitale and is the horizontal reference plane of the floor or, more relevant to dentistry, the articulator on the human with the patient sitting upright and looking out to the horizon. It is important not to create a cant in our restorations which is unaesthetic and disrupts function.

Axis – Orbital Plane (AOP) This is a line joining the condylar axis and the lower border of the orbit. This is another horizontal reference plane of an articulator on the human.

Curve of Spee If the lower anteriors have worn then this will need to be corrected. The lower occlusal plane in an anterior posterior direction is called the curve of Spee (Figure 15.14). Analysis of skulls suggested that the molar surfaces lie on an arc and became the basis of Monson's 1932 spherical theory on the ideal arrangement of teeth in the arch. The curve of Spee refers to an arc (part of a circle that on average is 4 in.) that is tangential to the incisal edges and the buccal tips of the mandibular dentition viewed in a sagittal plane as discussed in a review article by Kumar and Tamizharasi (2012); they suggested that the curve of Spee has biomechanical function during food processing by increasing the crush to shear ratio between the posterior teeth and the efficiency of occlusal forces during mastication.

Phonetics Please read Chapter 7 for an introduction. The restorative considerations are important and the use of phonetics allows us to analyse vertical dimension and incisal length.

Two letters provide information specific to incisal length:

- F – fifty five – the incisal edge should touch the lower lip slightly.
- E – EEEEE – the incisors occupy the space between the lips and a guide of 50–80% is desirable.

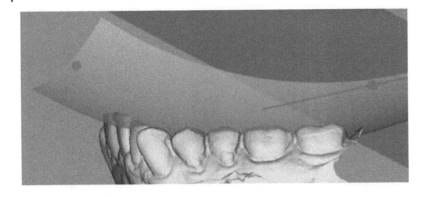

CURVE OF SPEE

Figure 15.14   Curve of Spee.

Two letters provide information specific to vertical dimension.

- S – sixty six – the teeth must not touch when articulating this sound.
- M – Emma – during articulation the interarch space is 2–4 mm.

Joint Loading and Sleep Apnoea   Please read Chapter 8.

Anterior Guidance   Please read Chapter 7.

Centric Relation
Please read Chapter 3.

Why are we using CR in TSL/TW? The main reason would be a CO that has failed or changed due to wear. We now need another reference point and we therefore use the joint. As we are increasing OVD in these cases, the arc of increase needs to be completed on an articulator. To ensure that we have a good representation of the articulatory system in the articulator, we also use a facebow. Accurate impressions for study casts are required ideally using silicone in rigid trays. For study cast examination and verification, see Chapter 3.

Dahl Concept

This method is used to restore localised anterior tooth wear. This is an anterior bite plane and previous methods used cobalt chrome removable appliances or cemented fixed prostheses but since the advent of adhesive materials, composite is the preferred choice. A systematic review by Ahmed and Murbay (2015) suggests survival rates of over 90% at 2.5 years and that separates the posterior teeth and therefore out of occlusion. The occlusal re-establishment is variable and in some individuals can take up to 24 months depending upon eruptive potential which cannot be measured; the review article states that increasing the OVD resulted in posterior occlusion re-establishment within 18 months for 91% of patients. If all the teeth do not come into contact, then we can simply add composite and provide occlusal proprioception. This method reduces the number of teeth being treated and is minimally invasive. However, in severe Class 3 skeletal and incisal relationships it cannot be used.

Poyser et al. (2005) categorised adverse reactions.

- *Pulpal symptoms* – these are rare and ultimately pulpal health is already compromised due to the wear. Therefore if root canal treatment is required, it will most likely have been due to extensive wear rather than the composite additions, but occlusal management is important to ensure equal distribution of the forces.
- *Periodontal symptoms* – patients can have some initial tenderness, but this generally resolves. The periodontal condition must be stable. The teeth can be splinted to reduce mobility but the shallowing of the incisal guidance and improving the axial forces as shown in Figure 15.6 are important in reducing unwanted forces and movement.
- *Speech and chewing* – chewing is initially unusual and awkward and lisping can occur.
- *Temporomandibular joint symptoms* – the literature has reported postoperative tenderness and muscle fatigue but all were transient and no long-term issues remained.

We need to be careful with Class 2 skeletal relationships with a large horizontal slide. The risk is distalising the mandible and losing anterior guidance which can also cause posterior rotation which can affect the airway and increase sleep apnoea.

How much space do we need for the material and therefore how much do we increase the OVD? Two factors dictate this.

- *Function* – bulk thickness and strength of the material – composite needs a minimum 1.5 mm.
- *Aesthetics* – incisal visibility at rest with incisor proportion measurements. If there is 2 mm or more of incisal visibility at rest, we cannot add more material to the incisors so we must then lift the gum (crown lengthening) to increase incisal length (Figure 15.15).

Methods used to analyse increase in OVD are as follows (this is addressed in greater detail in Chapter 17).

- Measurement of CEJ to CEJ.
- Facial proportions (described above).
- Trial appliances such as splints, orthotics, etc.
- Freeway space.
- Rest position obtained using a transcutaneous electrical nerve stimulation (TENS) appliance.
- Phonetics – 'M' and 'S'.

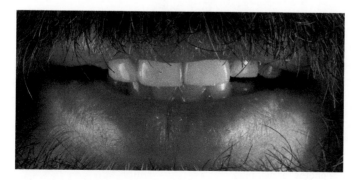

Figure 15.15   Incisal visibility at rest.

This forms the basis for an aesthetic wax-up and can be transferred as a mock-up allowing a smile preview.

This completes the consent process and we now can test:

- aesthetics
- phonetics
- occlusion.

Steps for DAHL Treatment

1) Checklist as above – using photographs.
2) Accurate articulated records – study models, CR registration record, facebow with preoperative occlusal records.
3) Aesthetic and functional wax-up – static stops on cingulum platforms. Canine guidance and protrusive guidance on central incisors.
4) Transfer to the patient – postoperative occlusal records.
5) Monitor – every 3 months, repeating occlusal measurements.

Stages.

1) Photographs required Figure 15.16 illustrates the photographs required for planning..

- Full face – frontal and with retracted view
- Incisal view at rest
- Smiling photo
- Intraoral pictures – frontal, lateral and occlusal views

2) Measurements required.

- Maxillary and mandibular central incisors view at rest
- Width and length of central incisor – mandibular and maxillary

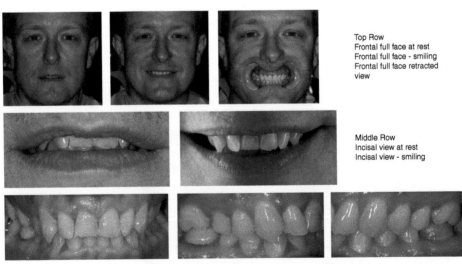

Top Row
Frontal full face at rest
Frontal full face - smiling
Frontal full face retracted view

Middle Row
Incisal view at rest
Incisal view - smiling

Bottom Row - Intraoral frontal view, Intraoral right lateral view, Intraoral left lateral view,

Figure 15.16   Preoperative case photos for planning.

- Overjet, overbite, and OVD
- Amount of space between CR and CO
- Choice of material

This dictates where we place the material. Figure 15.17 illustrates the options.
3) Laboratory prescription – this will dictate the increase in OVD.
4) Preoperative occlusal contacts – shimstock holds.
5) Transfer to the mouth – there are numerous techniques but that is beyond the scope of this book.
6) Postoperative occlusal checks – anterior teeth – static contacts on all six teeth; dynamic contacts – canine guidance and protrusive guidance on central incisors.
7) Review appointments every 12 weeks – check static and dynamic contacts and shimstock holds until all teeth are in contact.
8) Stabilisation splint fabrication once teeth are in contact if cause of attrition is parafunction.

Measurements required.
1) Maxillary central incisor visibility at rest – 3 mm.
2) Maxillary central incisor width and length – 7.5×8.5 mm = 88%. An increase of 1 mm in length gives 78% proportionality. This also increases the visibility at rest to 4 mm (within the normal range).
3) Overjet – 1 mm.
   Overbite 3 mm.
   OVD – 16 mm CEJ of canine.

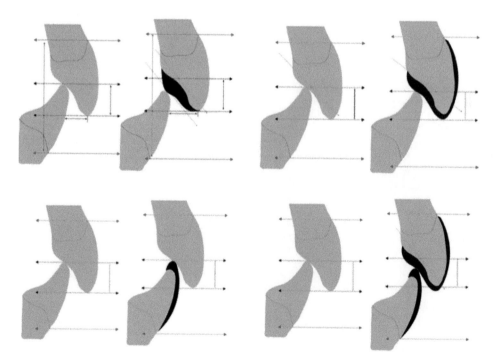

Figure 15.17   Illustrating the options where material can be placed once an increase in OVD is determined.

4) The amount of space between CR and CO – first tooth contact – provided 0.5 mm.
5) Choice of material – composite (hybrid filler particles recommended). Minimum thickness for composite is 1.5 mm.
6) Shimstock holds preoperative record.

The required OVD increase is 2 mm in this case to provide enough bulk of material and improve the aesthetics by increasing the length of the central incisors by 1 mm.

Laboratory Prescription

Articulate models in centric relation using facebow record and CR registration record.

Wax up upper right canine to upper left canine palatal aspect and labial of central and lateral incisors. Increase central incisal length by 1 mm.

OVD increase is 2 mm using CEJ of the upper and lower right canines. Increase the vertical pin by 3 mm.

This is the 'rule of thirds'. An increase in the vertical pin at 3 mm equates to a 2 mm increase in the incisor region and 1 mm increase on the molars as shown by Rebibo et al. (2009). This is a guide because positioning the study cast within the articulator allows for correct arc of closure but if the model is too close to the vertical pin then this rule is not accurate (Figure 15.18).

Clinical stages and the numerous techniques that can be used to transfer the wax-up to the mouth are not dealt with in this book. Milosevic (2018) provides an evidence-based approach when using composite to restore worn teeth with clinical steps.

The occlusion needs assessing postoperatively (Figures 15.19–15.22). This will be monitored until space closure and shimstock holds are re-established.

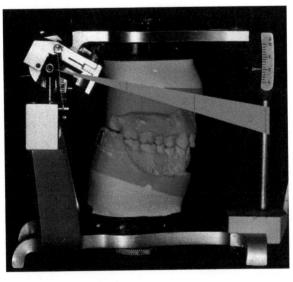

RULE OF "THE THIRDS";
for a
3 mm increase at incisal pin,
we obtain a 2 mm increase
on incisors and 1 mm
increase on Molars

Figure 15.18   Rule of thirds.

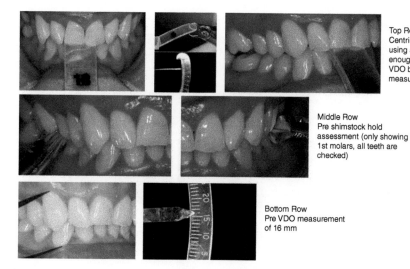

Top Row
Centric relation record taken
using a leaf gauge with
enough leaves to increase
VDO by 2 mm. Leaf gauge
measured using callipers

Middle Row
Pre shimstock hold
assessment (only showing
1st molars, all teeth are
checked)

Bottom Row
Pre VDO measurement
of 16 mm

Figure 15.19   CR record and clinical steps and assessment.

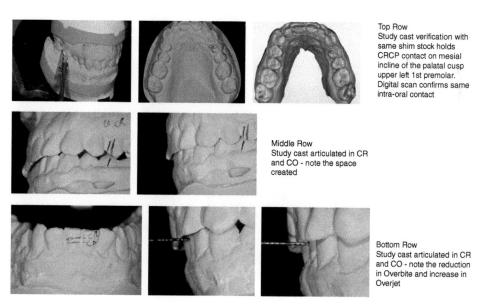

Top Row
Study cast verification with
same shim stock holds
CRCP contact on mesial
incline of the palatal cusp
upper left 1st premolar.
Digital scan confirms same
intra-oral contact

Middle Row
Study cast articulated in CR
and CO - note the space
created

Bottom Row
Study cast articulated in CR
and CO - note the reduction
in Overbite and increase in
Overjet

Figure 15.20   Laboratory steps and assessment.

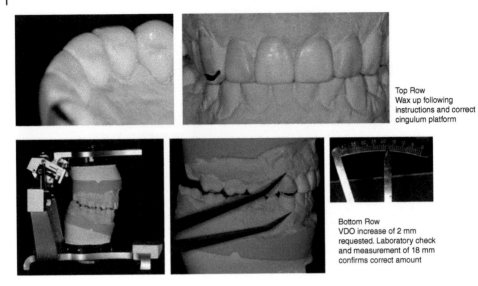

Top Row
Wax up following
instructions and correct
cingulum platform

Bottom Row
VDO increase of 2 mm
requested. Laboratory check
and measurement of 18 mm
confirms correct amount

Figure 15.21   Laboratory wax-up and assessment.

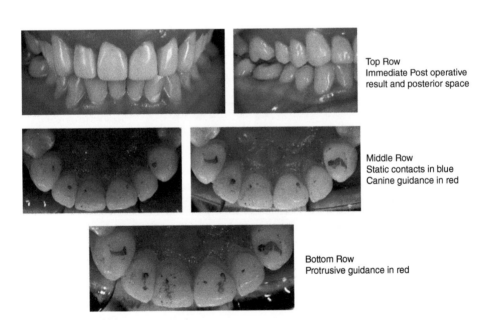

Top Row
Immediate Post operative
result and posterior space

Middle Row
Static contacts in blue
Canine guidance in red

Bottom Row
Protrusive guidance in red

Figure 15.22   Postoperative result.

References

Addy, M. and Shellis, R.P. (2006). Interaction between attrition, abrasion and erosion in tooth wear. *Monogr. Oral Sci.* 20: 17–31.

Ahmed, K.E. and Murbay, S. (2015). Survival rates of anterior composites in managing tooth wear: systematic review. *J. Oral Rehabil.* 43: 145–153.

Bartlett, D.W., Evans, D.F., Anggiansah, A., and Smith, B.G. (1996). A study of the association between gastro-oesophageal reflux and palatal dental erosion. *Br. Dent. J.* 181: 125–131.

Carvalho, T.S., Colon, P., Ganss, C. et al. (2016). Consensus report of the European Federation of Conservative Dentistry: erosive tooth wear diagnosis and management. *Swiss. Dent. J.* 126: 342–346.

Crothers, A. and Sandham, A. (1993). Vertical height differences in subjects with severe dental wear. *Eur. J. Orthod.* 15 (6): 519–525.

Cuniberti, N. and Rossi, G. (2019). Abfraction – myth or reality? Why some wedge-shaped cervical lesions are not caused by acid erosion. *Int. J. Dent. Oral Health.* 6 (1): 1–8.

Dahl, B.L., Krogstad, O., and Karlsen, K. (1975). An alternative treatment in cases with advanced localized attrition. *J. Oral Rehabil.* 2: 209–214.

Davies, S.J., Gray, R.J.M., and Qualtrough, A.J.E. (2002). Management of tooth surface loss. *Br. Dent. J.* 192: 11–23.

Grippo, J.O., Simring, M., and Schreiner, S. (2004). Attrition, abrasion, corrosion and abfraction revisited. *JADA* 135: 1109–1118.

Jain, V., Mathur, V.P., and Kumar, A. (2013). A preliminary study to find a possible association between occlusal wear and maximum bite force in humans. *Acta Odontol. Scand.* 71 (1): 96–101.

Kumar, K.P. and Tamizharasi, S. (2012). Significance of curve of Spee: an orthodontic review. *J. Pharm. Bioallied Sci.* 4 (Suppl 2): S323–S328.

Lee, W.C. and Eakle, W.S. (1984). Possible role of tensile stress in the etiology of cervical erosion lesions in teeth. *J. Prosthet. Dent.* 52: 374–380.

Milosevic, A. (2018). Clinical guidance and an evidence-based approach for restoration of the worn dentition by direct composite resin. *Br. Dent. J.* 224 (5): 301–310.

Muts, E.J., van Pelt, H., Edelhoff, D. et al. (2014). Tooth wear: a systematic review of treatment options. *J. Prosthet. Dent.* 112: 752–759.

Pigno, M.A., Hatch, J.P., Rodrigues-Garcia, R.C. et al. (2001). Severity, distribution, and correlates of occlusal tooth wear in a sample of Mexican-American and European-American adults. *Int. J. Prosthodont.* 14 (1): 65–70.

Pindborg, J.J. (1970). *Pathology of the Dental Hard Tissues*, 1e, 294–321. Philadelphia: Saunders.

Poyser, N., Porter, R., Briggs, P. et al. (2005). The Dahl concept: past, present and future. *Br. Dent. J.* 198: 669–676.

Rebibo M, Darmouni L, Joivin J. Vertical dimension of occlusion: the keys to decision. *J. Stomat. Occ. Med.* 2009; 2: 147–159.

Ricketts, R. (2009). Planning treatment on the basis of the facial pattern and an estimate of its growth. *Angle Orthod.* 27: 14–37.

Stănuşi, A., Mercuţ, V., Scrieciu, M. et al. (2020). Analysis of stress generated in the enamel of an upper first premolar: a finite element study. *Stoma. Edu. J.* 7 (1): 28–34.

Tjan, A.H., Miller, G.D., and The, J.G. (1984). Some esthetic factors in a smile. *J. Prosthet. Dent.* 51 (1): 24–28.

Further Reading

Dahl, B.L. and Krogstad, O. (1982). The effect of a partial bite raising splint on the occlusal face height. An x-ray cephalometric study in human adults. *Acta Odontol. Scand.* 40: 17–24.

Mizrahi, B. (2006). The Dahl principle: creating space and improving the biomechanical prognosis of anterior crowns. *Quintessence International* 37(4): 245–51.

Monson, G.S. (1932). Applied mechanics to the theory of mandibular movements. *Dent. Cosmos.* 74: 1039–1053.

Spee, F.G. (1980). The gliding path of the mandible along the skull. *J. Am. Dent. Assoc.* 100: 670–675.

Sterrett, J.D., Oliver, T., Robinson, F. et al. (1999). Width/length ratios of normal clinical crowns of the maxillary anterior dentition in man. *J. Clin. Periodontol.* 26 (3): 153–157.

16

All My Teeth Are Restored But Don't Meet Like They Did Before

Scenario

The patient has presented with a restored mouth with multiple crowns and they feel the teeth do not meet like before. They cannot find a comfortable position (Figure 16.1).

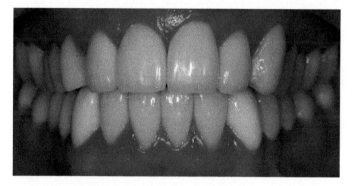

Figure 16.1   Clinical presentation of the patient.

Rationale

What is the risk of occlusal imprecision? Chapter 2 discusses the neuroanatomy and periodontal mechanoreceptors in detail. This is a feedback and feedforward system with inter-individual variations. Therefore, if we place a restoration or change the occlusion, risks exist but the view that the teeth alone are the root of all problems requires an expansive outlook and the use of certain terminology, such as interference or malocclusion, does not aid this process. The literature has delved into this topic; Clark et al. (1999) looked at 18 human and 10 animal occlusal interference studies and concluded that symptoms do occur such as transient local tooth pain, increased mobility, altered chewing patterns and muscle tension and occasional click and jaw pain but these arose in patients who had no previous temporomandibular disorder (TMD) issues. The studies do have limitations; the sample

Practical Procedures in Dental Occlusion, First Edition. Ziad Al-Ani and Riaz Yar.
© 2022 John Wiley & Sons Ltd. Published 2022 by John Wiley & Sons Ltd.
Companion website: www.wiley.com/go/al-ani-and-riaz/dental-occlusion

sizes were small, the largest group being 27, and the duration of the studies was short, the longest being 27 days.

Klineberg and Eckert (2015) state that there is a lack of understanding of the facts that:

1) the somatosensory input is continuously modulated by the central nervous system by means of descending mechanisms
2) the sensorimotor system is plastic, not hard wired (has the capacity to adapt to functional demand)
3) cognitive, affective and emotional factors often determine if and how a patient adjusts to dental treatment.

Point 3 is crucial to our understanding of the patient and the motivating factors for seeking treatment. The studies also provide two conclusions that affect the management of your patient.

1) There are individual differences in vulnerability to occlusal interferences.
2) Acute occlusal interferences may cause different symptoms, which in healthy individuals disappear within 1–2 weeks at most. It is therefore correct to reassure patients that they will adjust to the new reconstruction. However, longer lasting symptoms are a sign that either the reconstruction is incorrect or the dentist is managing a patient with poor adaptability (e.g. a patient at risk of developing an occlusal dysesthesia). Thus, one could hypothesise that the introduction of an occlusal interference could be a test to check the adaptability of a patient. This is a provocative statement, but it underlines the need for a paradigm shift in how dentists must look at the occlusion.

So What is Occlusal Dysthesia?

Defined by Hara et al. (2012), occlusal dysthesia is a persistent complaint of uncomfortable bite sensation for more than 6 months, which does not correspond to any physical alteration related to the occlusion, dental pulp, periodontium, jaw muscles or temporomandibular joints (TMJs). It is also known as a 'phantom bite' and is frequently associated with psychiatric conditions. This condition is rare with little prevalence data. Watanabe et al. (2015) surveyed 130 patients and found that 70% reported that symptoms developed after dental treatment.

The aetiology is unclear and there are three suggested mechanisms.

- *Psychopathological* – Marbach et al. (1983) described it as a delusional disorder that may have links with body dysmorphic disorder so the patients do not just complain about the bite but also that the teeth do not look right. Therefore, assessment to determine the current psychological state is important in dentistry. A public health questionnaire (PHQ-4) is an ultra-brief screener for anxiety and depression, and it is a valid tool as discussed by Kroenke et al. (2009). If the score indicates psychological distress, then referral to their general medical practitioner is advised before embarking on dental treatment.
- *Neuromatrix theory* – based on Melzack's (1999) theory that a matrix of neurons exists in the central nervous system, genetically predisposed and influenced by external stimuli; the output of those neurons is called the neurosignature, which represents the

self-knowledge of the whole body. Marbach related this to dentistry and coined the term 'occlusal neurosignature'; when dental treatments modify or alter this, it leads to a distorted interpretation of the changed bite and can cause occlusal dysthesia (OD) in predisposed subjects.

- *Altered dental proprioception* – this theory proposes that patients with OD have a higher or heightened sensitivity. Baba et al. (2005) conducted a thickness discrimination test and while patients with OD displayed better thickness discrimination ability than controls (8 vs 14 μm), the difference was not statistically significant. This is occlusal hypervigilance which is simply a by-product of the emotional state of patients with OD, but acts together with cognitive, behavioural and affective negativity in symptom causation and maintenance. It is more likely that patients misinterpret normal occlusal sensations (Table 16.1).

Diagnostic criteria have been suggested by Melis and Zawawi (2015).

- Complaint of uncomfortable bite sensation.
- Significant associated emotional distress.
- The symptoms last for more than 6 months.
- History of various bite-altering dental procedure failures.
- Absence of dental occlusal discrepancies or disproportional to the complaint.
- Not attributed to another disorder (dental pathology, muscle, TMJ, or neurological disorder).

Treatment and management of these patients involve obtaining a detailed history and thorough TMJ and occlusal examination to eliminate a true odontogenic cause for the history. This is paramount because we do not want to embark on irreversible restorative treatment and reorganise the occlusion because the new occlusal contacts will also be a problem for the patient. If restorative treatment is justified after a conscientious assessment, then this must be tested and occlusal precision is required.

Table 16.1   Typical symptoms mentioned by patients.

Presenting complaints or expressions
• My bite is not comfortable
• My bite is off
• I do not know where my teeth belong any more
• My jaws are not biting correctly
• I feel my bite is wrong, my jaws are always wandering around looking for a comfortable position
• My bite is uneven
Co-morbidities – these symptoms are not always isolated
• Parafunction
• Temporomandibular disorders
• Anxiety and depression
• Obsessive compulsive disorders
• Somatoform disorder

If your diagnosis is OD the treatment is categorised into four areas.

1) *Patient education* – communication is key. This requires a scrupulous explanation that teeth contacts change continuously depending on posture, head position and muscle tension so teeth touching unevenly can be considered normal, but this usually happens unconsciously.

2) *Psychotherapy* – Cognitive behavioural therapy is primarily focused on distracting the patient's attention away from their teeth.

3) *Pharmacotherapy* – if the PHQ-4 highlights anxiety and depression then medications that can help stabilise their mood may be justified.

4) *Oral appliance therapy* – anterior bite planes and soft bite guards are used to mask the perception of occlusal contacts whereas a stabilisation splint aims to provide equal static contacts and canine guidance which reduces muscle activity and protrusive guidance with no interference. The risk is that this method may increase the patient's attention. The advantage with a stabilisation splint is the reversibility and allowing a testing of the occlusal scheme. If the patient's symptoms resolve with the splint, then we must wait to see if the symptoms reappear after the splint therapy has ceased. The splint is restarted and if the symptoms resolve then this provides the rationale for further treatment.

Procedure

The patient presented after having 20 crowns placed on upper and lower second premolar to second premolar. The reason for the treatment was purely aesthetics but problems arose through the treatment. No provisional stage was tested. The patient developed symptoms similar to OD (Figure 16.2).

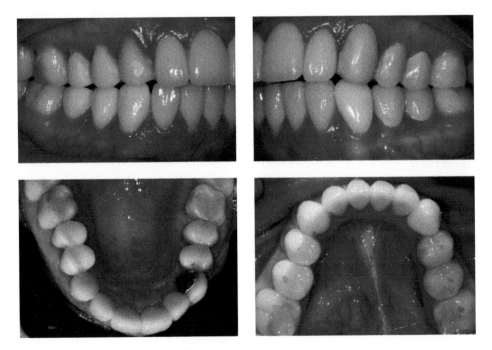

Figure 16.2 Preoperative clinical photographs.

Temporomandibular joint examination as detailed by Gray et al. (1995) confirmed myofascial pain and there were intraoral signs of cheek ridging and tongue scalloping which are signs of active parafunction. For a detailed TMJ analysis and rationale please see Chapter 9.

Temporomandibular Joint

Tender to palpation?	Lateral pole – tender left and right
	Intra-auricular – nothing abnormal detected (nad)

Noises	Clicks	Right, left or bilateral
		Soft or loud
		Consistent or intermittent
		Opening or closing or both
		Painful or painless
		Single or multiple
	Crepitus	Right, left or bilateral
		Painful or painless

Range of motion (mm)

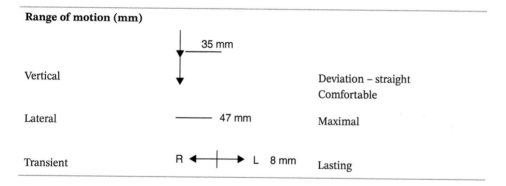

Vertical	35 mm	Deviation – straight
		Comfortable
Lateral	47 mm	Maximal
Transient	R ←—|—→ L 8 mm	Lasting

Muscle Tenderness

Temporalis	Origin and insertion – left and right tender	
Masseter	Origin and insertion – left and right tender	
Lateral pterygoid	nad	
Joint loading		
Right side	Myogenous	Arthrogenous – nad
Left side	Myogenous	Arthrogenous – nad
Signs of parafunction	Cheek ridging	Tongue scalloping
	Toothwear	Fractured teeth/restorations
Sleep Epworth score	4	

(Continued)

PHQ-4 score	4	
Occlusal examination	Skeletal	Class 2
	Incisal	Class 2 div 1
OVD – CEJ – CEJ	19 mm	
Overbite	Anterior open bite	
Overjet	8 mm	
Shimstock holds	17 47 27 37	

Static occlusion

Does CO occur in CR?	No
If not, where is CRCP exactly?	Mesial incline Mesiopalatal cusp 27
Direction of slide from CR	Small horizontal and vertical
Freedom in centric occlusion	Yes

Dynamic occlusion

	RHS	LHS
Canine guidance		
Group function	All guidance on 2nd molars	
NWS interference	27	17
WS interference	17	27

Treatment Plan

Phase 1 – stabilisation phase.

1) Occlusal splint – if successful, move to the restorative phase.

Phase 2 – provisionalisation phase.

1) Functional wax-up in centric relation (CR).
2) Transfer of wax-up.
3) Adjust and refine and test occlusal scheme – 8 weeks.
4) Only if long-term provisionals are required – impressions for laboratory-fabricated acrylic restorations.

Phase 3 – definitive treatment stage.

1) Posterior teeth – cross-mounting.
2) Anterior teeth.
3) Occlusal splint – post treatment.

Phase 1 – Stabilisation Phase

Occlusal examination allows for verification of the study casts, ensuring that the data captured intraorally also match when the study casts are articulated; therefore meticulous care is required when taking impressions. Alginate is used in rigid, ideally metal rimlock trays with adhesive but if multiple pours are required then silicone allows for this rather than using agar to duplicate the original study cast. For examination and verification of the study cast see Chapter 3.

An occlusal splint is defined by the GPT 2017 as 'any removable artificial occlusal surface used for diagnosis or therapy used for diagnosis or therapy affecting the relationship of the mandible to the maxilla. It may be used for occlusal stabilisation, for treatment of TMDs or to prevent wear of the dentition'. There are several names given to these splints.

- Stabilisation splint.
- CR splint.
- Michigan splint – a maxillary splint described by Ramjford and Ash and generally used in Class 1 and Class 2 cases.
- Tanner splint – a mandibular splint described by Henry Tanner and generally used in Class 3 cases.

The splint is full coverage to prevent iatrogenic tooth movement and is placed in the arch with teeth missing, allowing the opposing arch to provide greater proprioceptive feedback neurologically. Splint thickness should be between 3 and 5 mm ideally. The steps involved in occlusal splint fabrication are a facebow record (see Chapter 3), upper and lower arch impressions and CR record taken using a leaf gauge or Lucia jig or bimanual manipulation techniques. See Chapter 8 for laboratory stage.

Splint Usage Myofascial issues – treatment of muscle or joint pain especially from parafunction or to test occlusal discrepancies.

- Deprogramming of muscles to record CR.
- Vertical dimension alteration.

The splint is assessed for fit. If it is too tight then the internal aspects are adjusted and if too loose then they can be relined using a polymethylmethacrylate (PMMA) resin acrylic material such as Bosworth Trim® (Trim, Bosworth Co., USA).

Once stable, adjustments are required to ensure multiple stable intercuspal position (ICP) point contacts or centric stops from the supporting cusps and these should correspond to the same number of opposing teeth. Drying the splint using paper held in Miller's forceps and using 40 μm articulating paper allow for colour transfer. The acrylic bur is held parallel to the bite plane to ensure no fossa shapes are created causing resistance to lateral or protrusive movement. The anterior ramp provides immediate disclusion of the posterior teeth. The ramp must be shallow to reduce friction in lateral movements (Figure 16.3).

Occlusal plane discrepancies can make splint fabrication difficult and technically demanding.

Review and Wear Protocol The splint is generally worn at night only and the next review appointment is at 2–3 weeks. At the review appointment a history of symptoms is elicited; typically there is an improvement and the occlusal contacts are assessed. Due

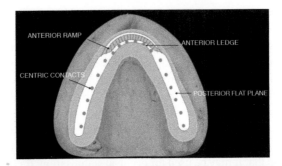

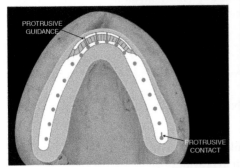

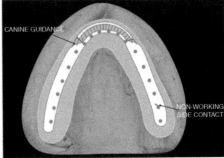

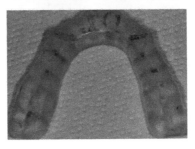

Figure 16.3   Stabilisation splint guidelines.

to a reduction in muscle tension and activity, the contacts will have changed, and further adjustments are required to reintroduce the original occlusal contacts. If symptoms have not changed then increasing the wear is an option and further reduction of the anterior ramp is provided. This review appointment is repeated typically four times until the occlusal contacts remain the same as the previous appointment and no adjustments are required.

Phase 2 – Provisionalisation Phase

This phase involves the use of prototypes to test the new occlusal scheme making centric occlusion (CO) and centric relation (CR) coincident. A facebow record, silicone arch impressions of the upper and lower arch with CR record are required (Figure 16.4).

A laboratory prescription for diagnostic wax-up is prescribed, stating a functional and aesthetic wax-up on all posterior teeth (Figure 16.5).

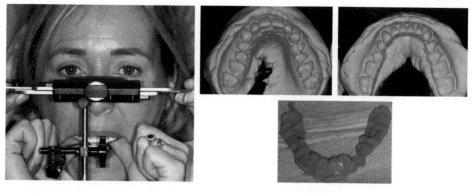

Figure 16.4   Clinical records stage.

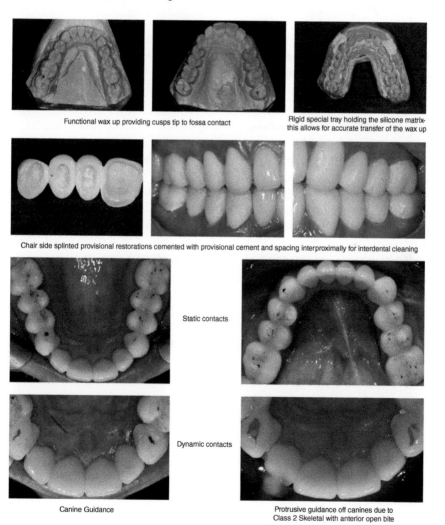

Functional wax up providing cusps tip to fossa contact

Rigid special tray holding the silicone matrix-this allows for accurate transfer of the wax up

Chair side splinted provisional restorations cemented with provisional cement and spacing interproximally for interdental cleaning

Static contacts

Dynamic contacts

Canine Guidance

Protrusive guidance off canines due to Class 2 Skeletal with anterior open bite

Figure 16.5   Provisionalisation stage.

Please articulate using facebow and CR record. Further information regarding CRCP is provided, for example 27 mesial incline of palatal cusp. A request for a silicone transfer is needed. For study cast verification please see Chapter 3.

The splinting of the provisional restoration and the reduced rigidity of the Bisacryl composite material may be sufficient in the majority of cases to test the occlusal scheme. The test phase period is 4–6 weeks as a minimum as discussed by Turner and Missirilian (1984). Symptoms that indicate the occlusal scheme is not appropriate for this patient include:

- repeated fracture of the provisional
- repeated debonding
- pulpitis symptoms
- muscular or joint pain.

Examine and adjust. Overjet and overbite should be analysed and ensure freedom in centric occlusion. See constricted chewing pattern in Chapter 15.

Some cases merit long-term provisionals depending on the history of symptoms and complexity of the case. The material of choice is PMMA.

Phase 3 – Transfer into Definitive Restorations

The information assimilated into the provisionals is very important in extensive rehabilitations. The optimal form (tooth shape and length, occlusal plane orientation, overbite, overjet, palatal morphology of the maxillary anterior teeth, angulation of the guiding inclines, vertical dimension of occlusion, teeth contacting) is not lost and is incorporated into the definitive restorations. There are different methods that can be used when completing this stage and the number of restorations that can be delivered to ensure occlusal precision. Once static and dynamic contacts have been established and the patient has adapted, how do we transfer into the definitive while preserving the occlusal vertical dimension (OVD) contacts.

The literature discusses several methods that can be used when completing a full mouth rehabilitation.

Option 1
1) Replace the posterior restorations to ensure posterior stability.
2) Then replace the anterior restorations.

Option 2
1) Replace the anterior restorations to maintain anterior guidance.
2) Then replace the posterior restorations.

The author's preferred method is option 1 which also allows for accurate cross-mounting. In rehabilitations involving both arches, the impressions to be made are:
- prepared abutments in the maxillary arch
- prepared abutments in the mandibular arch

- maxillary provisionals
- mandibular provisionals.

The corresponding bite registrations to be made (all at the same OVD and in the same mandibular position) are between:

- facebow registration with patient-approved provisional and CR record
- maxillary prepared abutments and mandibular prepared abutments
- maxillary prepared abutments and mandibular provisionals *or*
- maxillary provisionals and mandibular prepared abutments.

Each registration is made once, assuming that the operator is able to guide the mandible in CR with reproducibility. Otherwise, it is suggested to make three registrations and check to see if at least two are identical, as defined by Lucia (1964).

Gracis (2003) explains the benefits of cross-mounting the models of the provisionals: 'It allows the technician to have two important benefits. First, he or she can visualise the space available on the occlusal and palatal aspects not just statically, but, more importantly, dynamically as well, since the provisional restorations have been functioning and (should) have been successfully integrated in the mouth. Second, the technician can create a customised incisal guide table that will allow recreation of the same disclusion angles present in the provisionals in the final rehabilitation without guesswork'.

Steps
1) Take a facebow of the patient-approved provisional.
2) Take a CR record of the patient-approved provisional (Figure 16.6).
3) Articulate the patient-approved provisional case.
4) Articulate the opposing mandibular cast (natural dentition or a cast of the provisionals).
5) Once the mandibular cast is articulated, then the cast of the maxillary preparations is mounted with a bite registration to the mandibular teeth or provisionals, again at the OVD.
6) The cast of the mandibular prepared teeth is now mounted to the cast of the maxillary preparations.

Laboratory stages (Figures 16.7 and 16.8).

Customised guidance table created by the provisional restorations (see Chapter 11) (Figure 16.9).

Definitive restorations (Figure 16.10).

Postoperative occlusal check (Figure 16.11).

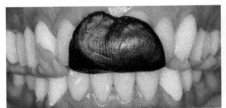

Green compound used an anterior stop to allow repeated closure into centric relation. Bite registration material placed on posterior teeth and allowed to set

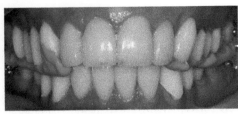

Green compound removed

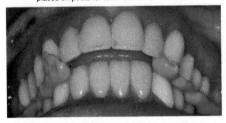

Note the open bite

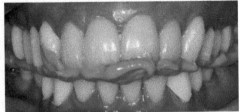

Bite registration record completed

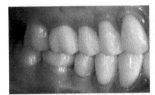

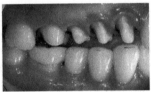

Provisionals

Maxillary prepared abutments against mandibular provisionals

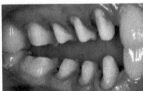

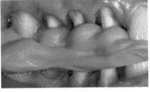

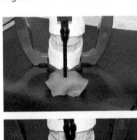

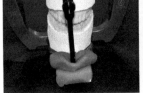

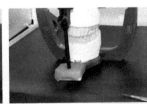

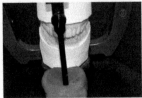

Maxillary prepared abutments against mandibular prepared abutments

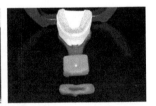

4 records -
1. Facebow record
2. CR record
3. Bite record - maxillary prepared abutments and mandibular provisionals
4. Bite record - maxillary prepared abutments and mandibular prepared abutments

Figure 16.6   Records for cross-mounting.

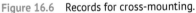

Top Row
Models articulated using face bow and CR record. The use of resin to fabricate the base of the incised guidance table

Middle Row
Resin Platform created and ready to carve the guidance from the provisionals

Figure 16.7   Customised incisal guidance table platform creation.

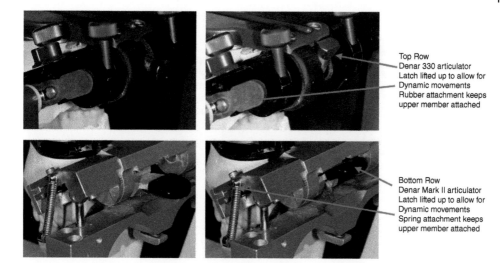

Top Row
Denar 330 articulator
Latch lifted up to allow for
Dynamic movements
Rubber attachment keeps
upper member attached

Bottom Row
Denar Mark II articulator
Latch lifted up to allow for
Dynamic movements
Spring attachment keeps
upper member attached

Figure 16.8   Articulator switch deactivated to allow lateral movements.

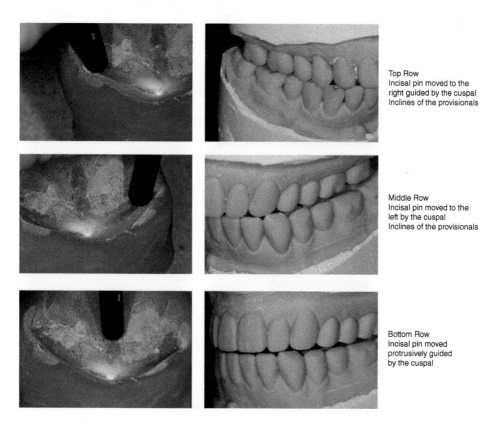

Top Row
Incisal pin moved to the
right guided by the cuspal
Inclines of the provisionals

Middle Row
Incisal pin moved to the
left by the cuspal
Inclines of the provisionals

Bottom Row
Incisal pin moved
protrusively guided
by the cuspal

Figure 16.9   Incisal guidance table – lateral movements.

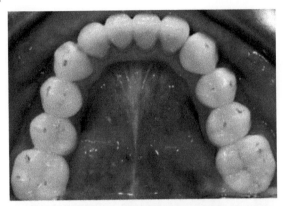

Top Row
Immediate Post operative
static contacts - note
anteriors have no contact
due to AOB

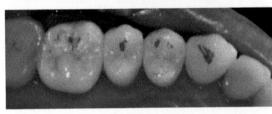

Middle Row
Immediate Post operative
dynamic contacts left side

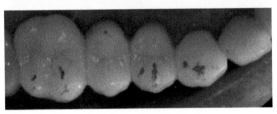

Bottom Row
Immediate Post operative
dynamic contacts right side

Figure 16.10   Final restorations.

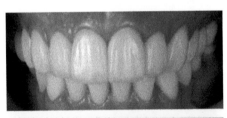

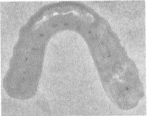

Post operative result with
final stabilisation splint

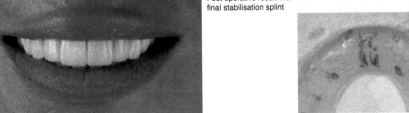

Figure 16.11   Anterior final restorations and post stabilisation splint.

References

Baba, K., Aridome, K., Haketa, T. et al. (2005). Sensory perceptive and discriminative abilities of patients with occlusal dysesthesia. *J. Jpn. Prosthodont. Soc.* 49: 599–607.

Clark, G.T., Tsukiyama, Y., Baba, K., and Watanabe, T. (1999). Sixty-eight years of experimental occlusal interference studies: what have we learned? *J. Prosthet. Dent.* 82 (6): 704–713.

Gracis, S. (2003). Clinical considerations and rationale for the use of simplified instrumentation in occlusal rehabilitation. Part 2: setting of the articulator and occlusal optimization. *Int. J. Periodontics Restorative Dent.* 23: 139–145.

Gray, R., Davies, S., and Quayle, A.A. (1995). *A Clinical Guide to Temporomandibular Disorders*. London: British Dental Journal.

Hara, E.S., Matsuka, Y., Minakuchi, H. et al. (2012). Occlusal dysesthesia: a qualitative systematic review of the epidemiology, aetiology and management. *J. Oral Rehabil.* 39: 630–638.

Klineberg, I. and Eckert, S. (2015). *Functional Occlusion in Restorative Dentistry and Prosthodontics*. St Louis, MO: Mosby.

Kroenke, K., Spitzer, R.L., Williams, J.B., and Löwe, B. (2009). An ultra-brief screening scale for anxiety and depression: the PHQ-4. *Psychosomatics* 50 (6): 613–621.

Lucia, V.O. (1964). A technique for recording centric relation. *J. Prosthet. Dent.* 14: 492–505.

Marbach, J.J., Varoscak, J.R., Blank, R.T., and Lund, P. (1983). "Phantom bite": classification and treatment. *J. Prosthet. Dent.* 49: 556–559.

Melis, M. and Zawawi, K.H. (2015). Occlusal dysesthesia: a topical narrative review. *J. Oral Rehabil.* 42 (10): 779–785.

Melzack, R. (1999). From the gate to the neuromatrix. *Pain* (suppl 6): S121–S126.

Turner, K. and Missirilian, D. (1984). Restoration of the extremely worn dentition. *J. Prosthet. Dent.* 52: 467–474.

Watanabe, M., Umezaki, Y., Suzuki, S. et al. (2015). Psychiatric comorbidities and psychopharmacological outcomes of phantom bite syndrome. *J. Psychosom. Res.* 78: 255–259.

Further Reading

Ramfjord, S.P. and Ash, M. (1994). Reflections on the Michigan occlusal splint. *J. Oral Rehabil.* 21 (5): 491–500.

17

I Am Breaking My Teeth and Veneers and Lost a Tooth Due to Grinding

Scenario

The patient has presented with generalised tooth wear. The teeth are occasionally sensitive and the patient is embarrassed to smile as previously applied veneers keep breaking and chipping off. They struggle to eat certain foods due to the fragile nature of their teeth and recently lost the lower left first molar due to a vertical fracture (Figure 17.1).

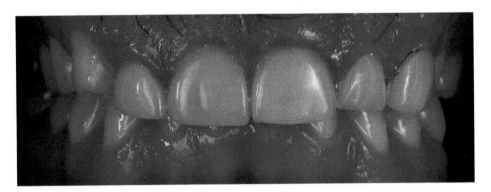

Figure 17.1   Patient presenting with chipped and lost veneers related to occlusal instability.

Rationale

Treatment planning is crucial and the three pilars of planning are desirability, suitability and affordability.

- *Desirability* – understanding the patient's desires right at the start allows the creation of a checklist and highlights whether their expectations are realistic and can be matched with suitability. The most common patient requirements are:
  - aesthetic – improvement of the smile
  - function – improvement of chewing
  - predictability/longevity – restorations not fracturing or coming out.

Practical Procedures in Dental Occlusion, First Edition. Ziad Al-Ani and Riaz Yar.
© 2022 John Wiley & Sons Ltd. Published 2022 by John Wiley & Sons Ltd.
Companion website: www.wiley.com/go/al-ani-and-riaz/dental-occlusion

- *Suitability* – an extra- and intraoral assessment with photographs and special investigations allows for detailed analysis of the environment in which we will place restorations.
- *Affordability* – presenting several options provides choice and allows the patient to make the right decision for their mouth.

To simplify, there are three options but sometimes not all are possible

- *Option 1, best advice* – this is the best advice the dentist can provide with regard to function, aesthetics, predictability and longevity.
  - Financial – requires a significant level of investment.
  - Materials – use of materials that are stronger and aesthetically pleasing such as ceramics.
  - Timeline – will involve lengthy appointments and an treatment extended schedule.

- *Option 2, compromise option* – this is a compromise in function, aesthetics, predictability and longevity. It will typically involve using materials that require a lower level of investment such as composite and therefore require greater maintenance.
- *Option 3, minimum option* – this option is the minimum that a clinician can offer to their patient.

The objective is to design a new smile that satisfies the patient's aesthetic and functional needs with correct biomechanical parameters.

Digital Occlusion

This is revolutionising dentistry and transforming our analysis of our patients. Analogue methods require the patient to fit the articulator but utilising digital technology, we can accurately transfer jaw movement data and incorporate this within the design of the restorations (Table 17.1).

The pioneers of this technique are Lundeen and Gibbs who between 1974 and 1985 developed the gnathic replicator to analyse jaw movement during mastication. Earlier devices such as the Denar Cadiax® or Arcus Digma™ are digital pentagraph systems designed for registration and display of mandibular hinge axis movements with data used to program the articulator and do not accurately represnt the human temporomandibular joint. The technology has evolved with the latest device entitled MODJAW developed by Maxime Jaisson using 4D data capture.

Table 17.1 Methods of analysing occlusion.

Analysis	Analogue	Digital
Static movement	Articulators	Digital articulators
Dynamic movement	Denar Cadiax	MODJAW
Occlusal contacts	Articulating paper	T-Scan
Facial aesthetics	Photographs	3D face scanning

The study casts are replaced with optical scanning which provides accurate images of the intraoral environment. Digital articulators are present within the digital software programs and can be set to the average values already in use with analogue devices. Articulating paper simply transfers colour but provides limited data with regard to force or timing of the contact while the use of digital analysis, initially discussed by Maness et al. (1987), features real-time force measurements recorded by the first T-Scan™ intraoral sensor.

Precision and attention to detail are still required to deliver accurate restorations.

Occlusal Vertical Dimension

In this case there is a requirement to increase the vertical dimension. In Chapter 15, the management of localised tooth wear utilising the Dahl concept involved increasing the vertical dimension but the primary reason for doing so was to restore lost tooth material by an additive technique. In this case, the posterior teeth are not worn so there is not a true loss of occlusal vertical dimension (OVD).

In generalised wear cases, the same principles apply except the posterior teeth are also worn and there is a true loss of OVD.

Understanding and managing OVD is important when extensive restorative treatment is required. The literature details several techniques.

- Measurement of cemento-enamel junction (CEJ) to CEJ.
- Facial proportions.
- Trial appliances such a splints, orthotics, etc.
- Freeway space.
- Rest position obtained using a transcutaneous electrical nerve stimulation (TENS) appliance.
- Phonetics – 'M' and 'S'.

Calamita et al. (2019) published a literature review of the techniques and history of each method. None of the techniques above has been shown to be sufficiently consistent and accurate to be used alone.

Tryde et al. (1977) also stated that OVD is not static and rigid but rather a vertical range of possible OVDs called the 'comfort zone'. This is why we must test the new OVD.

Three questions must be answered in order to manage OVD safely.

- Rationale for changing OVD.
- Determining the amount of OVD required.
- Clinically performing the change.

Rationale for Changing OVD

The main indications are as follows.

- *Aesthetics* – balancing and creating harmony: anterior teeth exposure during smiling and rest. This is detailed in Chapter 15.
- *Biomechanical* – creating adequate restorative space. Increasing the OVD allows for control over occlusal morphology and required thickness of the final restorative material but

more importantly we can bond to enamel. Therefore, the use of an additive adhesive mock-up allows the clinician to evaluate the patient's adaptability. Adjustments can be completed in this stage before delivering the definitive restorations.

- *Improving incisal and occlusal relationships* – when increasing the OVD, we alter the incisal relationship and this has an effect on the functional pathways and direction of the loads on teeth.
    - Static aspect – increase overjet and reduce overbite.
    - Dynamic aspect – phonetics and incisional guidance.

Determining the Amount of OVD Required (Figures 17.2 and 17.3)

This depends upon the skeletal relationship because an OVD increase can improve or worsen the arch relationship.

- Class 2 – worsen.
- Class 3 – compensation.

As a guide – 1 mm increase in incisal pin = 0.6 mm anterior space (0.6 mm overbite decrease and 0.4 mm overjet increase) and 0.3 mm posterior space and maintain same incisal guidance angle.

The amount required is ideally up to 5 mm as this is the safest amount. This case was increased 4 mm on the incisal pin. This provided anterior space of 2.6 mm and posterior space of 1.3 mm.

In the anterior space the overbite was reduced by 2 mm and overjet increased by 1.6 mm.

Biomechanically, the amount of additive material on both upper and lower incisors equated to 1.4 mm and posteriorly on the molars 0.65 mm. During preparation, the minimum required amount of material for monolithic zirconia is 1 mm therefore posteriorly, we

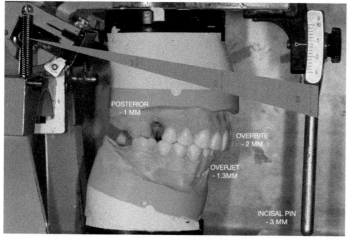

RULE OF "THE THIRDS";
for a
3 mm increase at incisal pin,
we obtain a 2 mm increase
on incisors and 1 mm
increase on
Molars

OVD increased by 3 mm on
incisal pin =
Anterior - 2 mm restorative
space
Overbite - reduced by 2 mm
Overjet increased by
1.3 mm
Posterior - increased 1 mm
restorative space

Figure 17.2   Articulated models detailing OVD increase with the 'rule of thirds'.

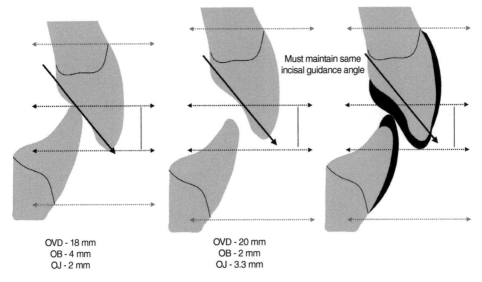

OVD - 18 mm
OB - 4 mm
OJ - 2 mm

OVD - 20 mm
OB - 2 mm
OJ - 3.3 mm

Must maintain same
incisal guidance angle

Figure 17.3   Diagrammatic illustration detailing increasing OVD.

would only be required to remove 0.35 mm of enamel and anteriorly no removal of enamel would be necessary. This is the reason why we increase the OVD. Our retention and resistance form are also improved. Occlusal planes are also corrected and non-working side contacts alleviated.

The incisal view at rest was 3 mm and the patient did not want to show any more. The width to length measurements are 7.5–8 mm therefore any changes to incisal length must involve lifting the gingivae using a crown lengthening procedure (Figure 17.4).

Is It Safe to Increase the OVD?

Abduo (2012) concluded that an increase of up to 5 mm is safe and without detrimental consequences and any associated signs and symptoms are self-limiting with a tendency to resolve within 2 weeks. There are no long-lasting effects on the Temporomandibular joint (TMJ), neuromuscular system, teeth, or phonetics as long as the interocclusal contacts are bilateral, simultaneous with axial loads, and the anterior teeth permit adequate phonetics and path of closure. Yabushita et al. (2006) and numerous other authors concluded that there is a reduction in masseter muscle spindle sensitivity and functional plasticity just 5 days after OVD increase and similar results at 8 weeks.

Conclusion Regarding OVD

There is a great capacity for adaptation in changing the OVD but three points are critical.

- Increase in centric relation.
- Do not worsen a vertical skeletal type already out of standard.
- Preserve labial contact.

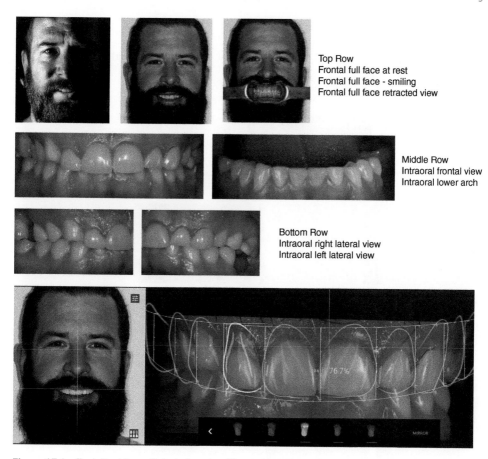

Top Row
Frontal full face at rest
Frontal full face - smiling
Frontal full face retracted view

Middle Row
Intraoral frontal view
Intraoral lower arch

Bottom Row
Intraoral right lateral view
Intraoral left lateral view

Figure 17.4   Facially driven digital planning. The smile design program Smilecloud highlights the discrepancy between width and length, delivering a 77% proportion.

Procedure

Silicone indexes are used to transfer to the mouth and trial the smile and aesthetics – labial wax transfer (Figures 17.5 and 17.6).

The smile preview is a crucial stage, which allows determination of shade acceptance, incisal visibility and shapes preview. Once approved, the full wax-up can be transferred (Figure 17.7).

Aesthetic Analysis

- Smile and incisal view at rest.
- Patient feedback regarding the shade and shape.

Functional Analysis

- Phonetics – performed while recording a video.
- Feedback from patient regarding mastication.

The final mock-up is then assessed (Figure 17.8).

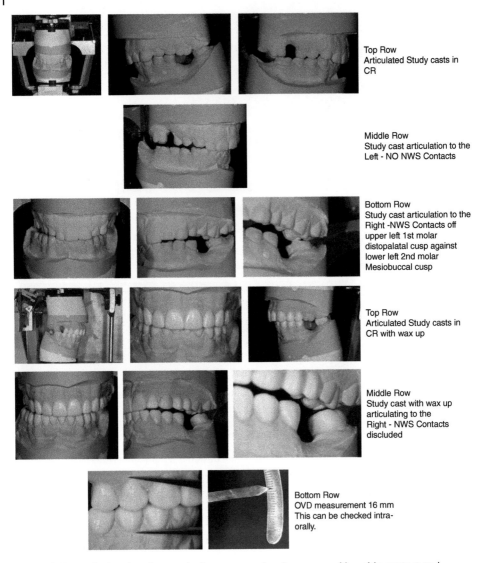

Top Row
Articulated Study casts in CR

Middle Row
Study cast articulation to the Left - NO NWS Contacts

Bottom Row
Study cast articulation to the Right -NWS Contacts off upper left 1st molar distopalatal cusp against lower left 2nd molar Mesiobuccal cusp

Top Row
Articulated Study casts in CR with wax up

Middle Row
Study cast with wax up articulating to the Right - NWS Contacts discluded

Bottom Row
OVD measurement 16 mm This can be checked intra-orally.

Figure 17.5 Articulated study casts before wax-up showing non-working side contact and occlusal plane.

Digital Scanning

There is no requirement for a customised incisal guidance table or facebow when digital scanning is used. A biocopy scan is taken which is a copy of the provisional tested occlusion (Figures 17.9 and 17.10). This is imported and duplicated in the digital design.

Postocclusal Analysis Utilising the T-Scan

The T-Scan state-of-the-art digital technology helps clinicians to identify premature contacts, high forces and interrelationship of occlusal surfaces. These important data cannot be captured by traditional, analogue occlusal methods, like articulating paper.

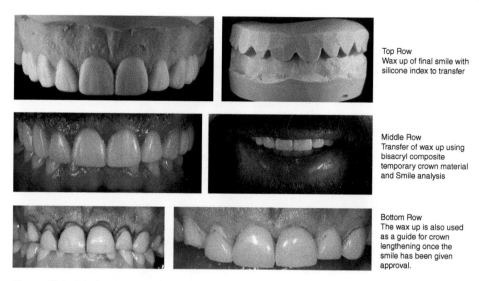

Top Row
Wax up of final smile with silicone index to transfer

Middle Row
Transfer of wax up using bisacryl composite temporary crown material and Smile analysis

Bottom Row
The wax up is also used as a guide for crown lengthening once the smile has been given approval.

Figure 17.6   Mock-up smile preview.

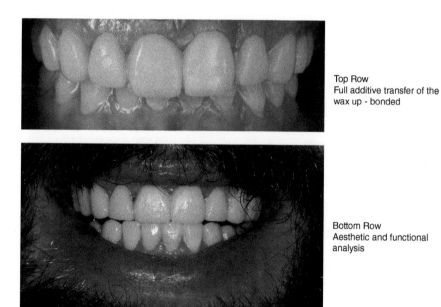

Top Row
Full additive transfer of the wax up - bonded

Bottom Row
Aesthetic and functional analysis

Figure 17.7   Functional mock-up transferred.

Whether eliminating destructive forces on a new restoration or performing an occlusal analysis and adjustment procedure, a T-Scan helps you balance your patient's occlusion. The T-Scan sensor allows for pressure mapping (Figure 17.11).

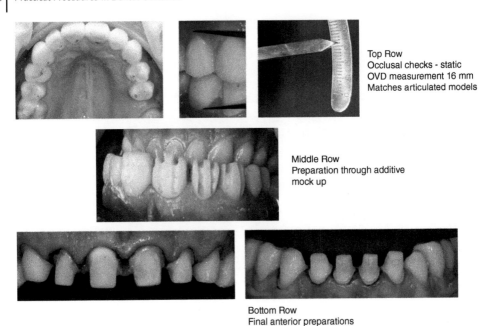

Top Row
Occlusal checks - static
OVD measurement 16 mm
Matches articulated models

Middle Row
Preparation through additive
mock up

Bottom Row
Final anterior preparations

Figure 17.8   Mock-up preassessment allowing for preparation through the added material.

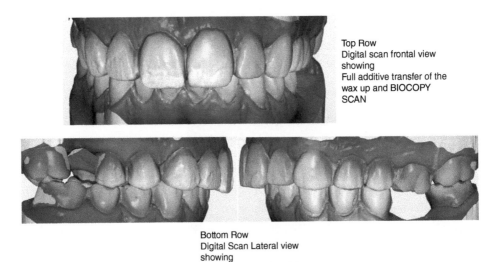

Top Row
Digital scan frontal view
showing
Full additive transfer of the
wax up and BIOCOPY
SCAN

Bottom Row
Digital Scan Lateral view
showing
Full additive transfer of the
wax up and BIOCOPY
SCAN

Figure 17.9   Digital biocopy scan to allow duplication into definitive restorations.

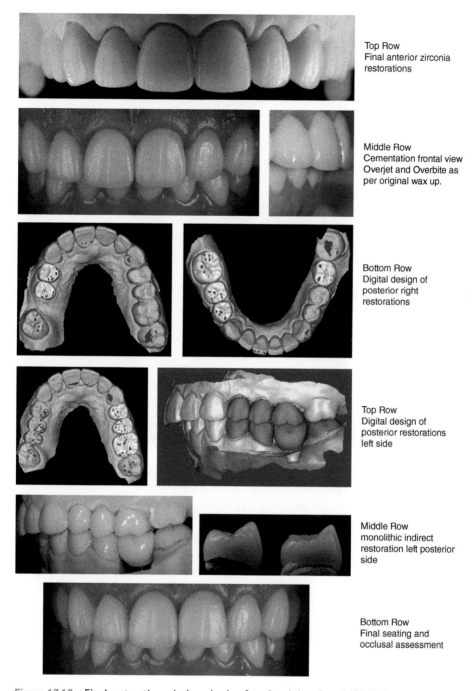

Top Row
Final anterior zirconia
restorations

Middle Row
Cementation frontal view
Overjet and Overbite as
per original wax up.

Bottom Row
Digital design of
posterior right
restorations

Top Row
Digital design of
posterior restorations
left side

Middle Row
monolithic indirect
restoration left posterior
side

Bottom Row
Final seating and
occlusal assessment

Figure 17.10   Final restorations designed using functional data from MODJAW.

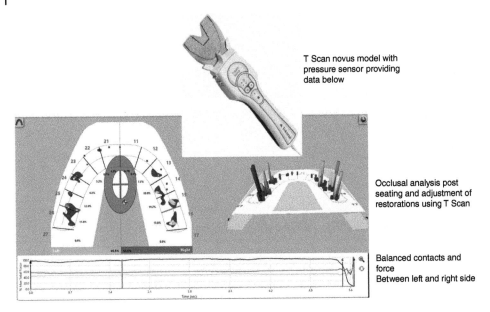

T Scan novus model with pressure sensor providing data below

Occlusal analysis post seating and adjustment of restorations using T Scan

Balanced contacts and force Between left and right side

Figure 17.11   T-Scan.

References

Abduo, J. (2012). Safety of increasing vertical dimension of occlusion: a systematic review. *Quintessence Int.* 43: 369–380.

Calamita, M., Coachman, C., Sesma, N., and Kois, J. (2019). Occlusal vertical dimension: treatment planning decisions and management considerations. *Int. J. Esthet. Dent.* 14: 166–181.

Maness, W.L., Benjamin, M., Podoloff, R. et al. (1987). Computerized occlusal analysis: a new technology. *Quintessence Int.* 18 (4): 287–292.

Tryde, G., Stoltze, K., Fujii, H., and Brill, N. (1977). Short-term changes in the perception of comfortable mandibular occlusal positions. *J. Oral Rehabil.* 4: 17–21.

Yabushita, T., Zeredo, L., Fujita, K. et al. (2006). Functional adaptability of jaw-muscle spindles after bite-raising. *J. Dent. Res.* 85: 849.

Further Reading

Lundeen, H.C., Shryock, E.F., and Gibbs, C.H. (1978). An evaluation of mandibular border movements: their character and significance. *J. Prosthet. Dent.* 40 (4): 442–452.

18

Occlusion on Implants. Any Difference?

Good Occlusal Practice in Implantology

While the roots and their periodontal ligaments (PDL) remain, mechanoreceptors allow finer discrimination of food texture, tooth contacts and levels of functional loading. This allows a better appreciation of food and a more precise control of mandibular movements than is provided by dental restorations.

The loss of periodontal mechanoreception around the dental implants means that there is no sensitive feedback from pulp or PDL. These restorations, therefore, react biomechanically in a different fashion to occlusal forces.

Studies have shown that the mean values of axial displacement of teeth in the socket vary between 25 and 100 µm. The range of motion of osseointegrated implants has been reported to be approximately 3–5 µm.

Dental implants may be more prone to occlusal overloading. The primary cause of peri-implantitis and bone loss around implants is the excessive force applied from unwanted occlusal contacts.

Moreover, patient adaptability is unpredictable at best and likely to be significantly reduced in implantology. The occlusal prescription of an implant-supported restoration, therefore, has to be much more carefully designed than that on a natural tooth.

The safest approach to adopt in implant dentistry is the 'conformative approach', that is to say, the occlusion of the implant-supported restoration should add to the existing occlusion but not change it.

Implant-Protected Occlusion (IPO): The Ten General Principles

Principle 1: Axial Loading is Required

Horizontal forces during chewing may cause potential damage or bone resorption around fixtures and should be avoided. Studies have shown that the cortical part of human long bones is strongest in compression, 30% weaker in tension and 65% weaker in shear.

Practical Procedures in Dental Occlusion, First Edition. Ziad Al-Ani and Riaz Yar.
© 2022 John Wiley & Sons Ltd. Published 2022 by John Wiley & Sons Ltd.
Companion website: www.wiley.com/go/al-ani-and-riaz/dental-occlusion

Therefore, the elimination or reduction of all shear loads to the implant system is mandatory because of the inherent weakness of bone – as well as porcelain, titanium components and cement – to shear loads (Figure 18.1).

Principle 2: Avoid Overloading Factors

Avoid overloading factors that may have a negative influence on implant longevity such as parafunctions, improper occlusal designs and premature contacts.

(a) (b)

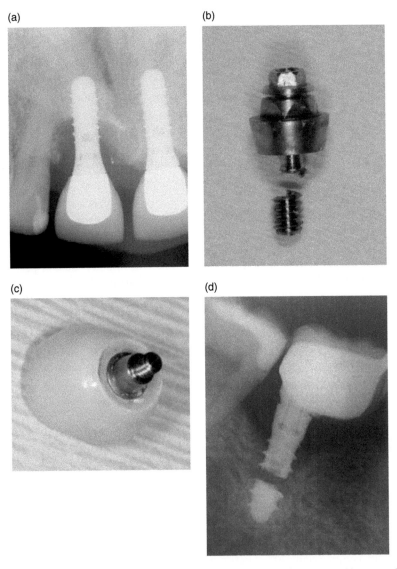

(c) (d)

Figure 18.1   (a) Bone loss (funnelling) around anterior implants caused by excessive occlusal forces. (b) Screw loosening, (c) abutment screw fractures, and (d) implant fractures may also occur from occlusal overload.

Principle 3: Implant Positioning

Orientation of the long axis of the fixture must be compatible with occluding elements. This generates masticatory forces parallel to each other. Any deviation from this norm will create components of horizontal force (compromise stability) (Figure 18.2).

Principle 4: Decrease Offset Loads

The ideal implant position is in line with the central fossa of the adjacent teeth. The supporting cusp of the opposing tooth must contact the element as close as possible to the axial centre of the abutment of the crown (Figure 18.3).

Centric stops should be centred over the central fossa, and secondary contacts may be placed greater than 1 mm from the marginal ridge (Figure 18.4).

Occlusal contacts on the cusp angles instead of the central fossa lead to an increase in the magnitude of shear stress on the implant and affect the physiological limit of compressive and tensile stress on the crestal bone (Figure 18.5).

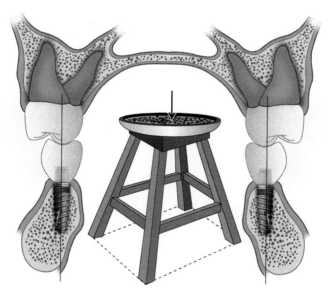

Figure 18.2　In implants, orient the total masticatory force loading to the force polygon principle.

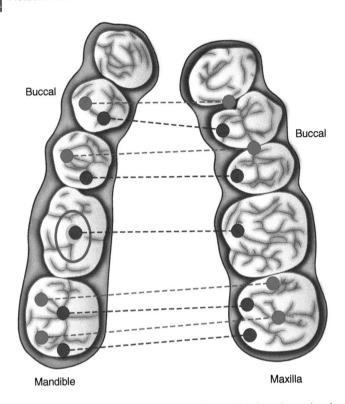

Buccal

Buccal

Mandible

Maxilla

Figure 18.3 Only one centric stop must be received on the occlusal surface of the implant.

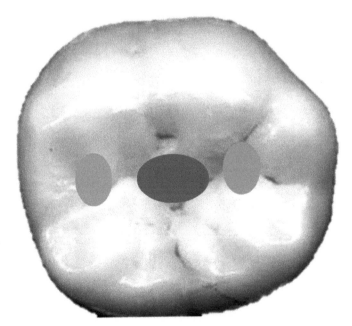

Figure 18.4 Centric stop (red) should be centred over central fossa, and secondary contacts (green) may be placed more than 1 mm from the marginal ridge. Marginal ridge contacts should be avoided.

Principle 5: Maintain a Narrow Posterior Occlusal Table

The cusp height should be reduced and the crown contour should ideally coincide with the diameter of the implant body. Normally, a 30–40% reduction in the occlusal table is recommended (Figure 18.6). In upper posterior implants, the occlusal table width should be decreased by reducing the palatal contour of the maxillary implant crown. This should ensure a decrease of offset loads on the implant (Figure 18.7). In contrast, in mandibular posterior implants, the buccal contour of the implant crown should be reduced (Figure 18.8).

When designing posterior implants, every attempt should be made to avoid extensive ridge lapping and cantilevers whenever possible. These designs have been considered as force magnifiers and a source of non-axial loading (Figure 18.9).

Maintaining the minimal posterior cusp inclination is also advocated when designing an implant-supported crown as large cusp angles create an increased contact surface area, resulting in shear forces. Flat cusps, however, result in concentrated forces over the implant body, thus reducing shear forces. Studies have shown that for every 10° increase in cusp inclination, a 30% increase in torque will result.

The clinician should adhere to a more shallow, or monoplane, cusp height, which will decrease force-related complications (Figure 18.10).

Principle 6: Freedom in Centric Concept Must Be Adopted

Centric platforms in the range of 2–3 mm for opposing supporting cusps must be created. This will minimise the possibility of premature contacts and allow for a more favourable force distribution (Figure 18.11).

Principle 7: Fine Tuning of the Occlusion

Fine adjustment of the occlusion in the form of slight infraocclusion should be adopted in implants occlusion. Ideally, a single anterior implant crown should have minimal contact during heavy occlusion and no contact on light occlusion.

Theoretically, many authors advise following a special protocol when designing implants; that is, in

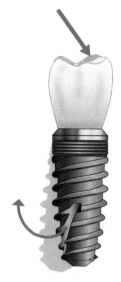

Figure 18.5 Occlusal contact on the cusp incline leads to an increase in the magnitude of shear stress around the implant.

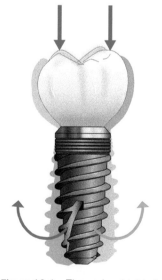

Figure 18.6 The occlusal table is too large, resulting in detrimental shear forces applied on the bone around the implant.

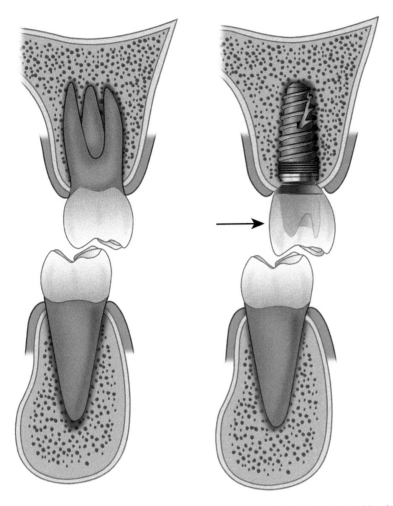

Figure 18.7 In an upper posterior implant, the occlusal table width should be decreased by reducing the palatal contour of the maxillary implant crown and the buccal cusp should have no occlusal contact.

centric occlusion the implant-supported crown should have a clearance of 30 μm in heavy clenching. The patient should be able to grip four layers of shimstock foil but three should pull through when they clench (refer to Chapter 3 for shimstock foil use) (Figure 18.12).

Principle 8: Increase Proximal Contact Area

A long, parallel proximal contact area allows for better force distribution between implants and natural teeth. An additional advantage is the ease of having one path of insertion for the prosthesis (Figure 18.13).

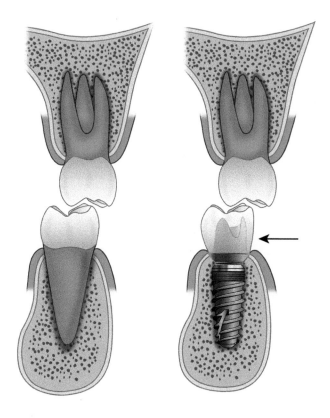

Figure 18.8   In a lower posterior implant, the buccal contour of the implant crown should be reduced.

Principle 9: Mutually Protected Articulation

No premature contacts on implant prostheses should be allowed and buccal and lingual cusps are shortened to avoid any gliding action against opposing teeth during lateral and protrusive excursions (Figure 18.14).

All excursive movements should be examined to make sure that disclusion of the proposed implant restorations with lateral excursions is carried by the existing natural teeth whenever possible (Figure 18.15).

In protrusive mandibular movements, the central and lateral incisors should disclude the posterior teeth (Figure 18.16).

Principle 10: Protection of Implants in Bruxists and Regular Evaluation and Maintenance

It is highly recommended to protect implant-supported restoration in patients with bruxism. Occlusal relationships of implants should be regularly evaluated, and accurate

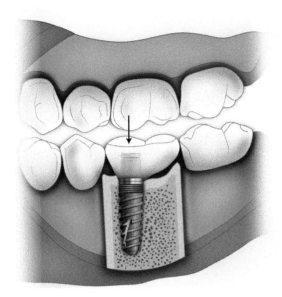

Figure 18.9   If the abutment of the implant crown is mesially or distally located in relation to its mesiodistal dimension, the opposing supporting cusp must make one contact on the occlusal surface of the crown in line with the axial alignment of the implant.

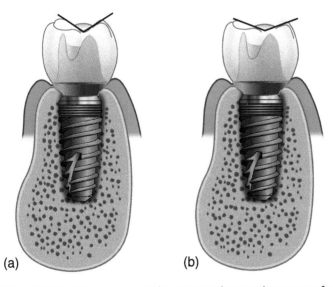

(a)   (b)

Figure 18.10   (a) Large cusp angles create an increased contact surface area, resulting in shear forces. (b) A more ideal flat cusp results in concentrated forces over the implant body, therefore reducing shear forces.

Figure 18.11   Freedom in centric concept must be adopted in posterior implants. Centric platforms in the range of 2–3 mm for opposing supporting cusps must be created.

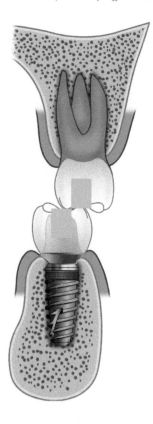

(a)   (b)

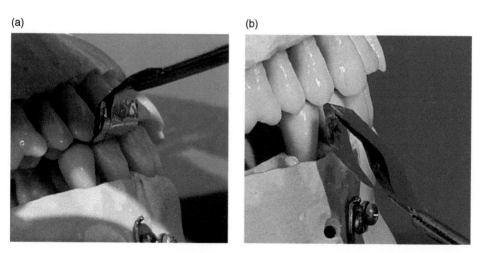

Figure 18.12   A suggested protocol in implant dentistry. In centric occlusion, the patient should be able to grip four layers of shimstock foil (a) but three should pull through when they clench (b) (refer to Chapter 3 for shimstock foil use).

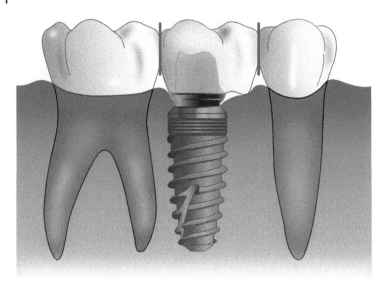

Figure 18.13 A long, parallel proximal contact area is recommended for better force distribution between implants and natural teeth.

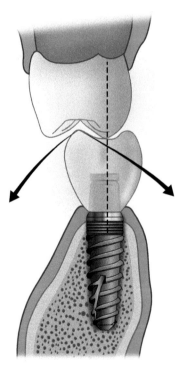

Figure 18.14 Buccal and lingual cusps are shortened to avoid any gliding action against the opposing tooth during lateral and protrusive excursions.

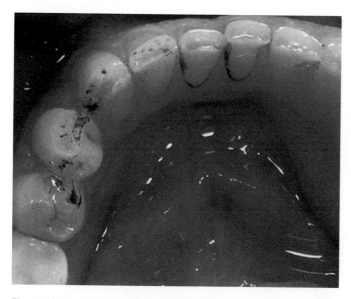

Figure 18.15   An ideal anterior guidance for an implant on a lower six. In this example, there is group function with no posterior interferences.

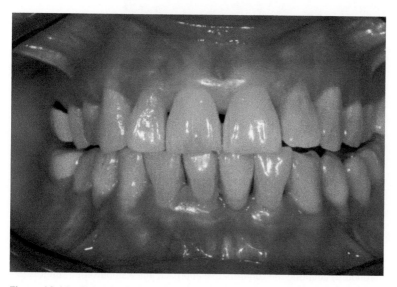

Figure 18.16   Posterior implant-supported restorations should be discluded during protrusive movement.

(a)

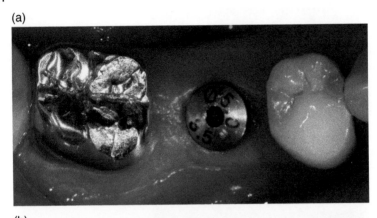

(b)

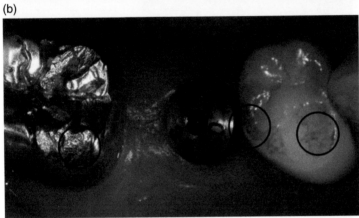

(c)

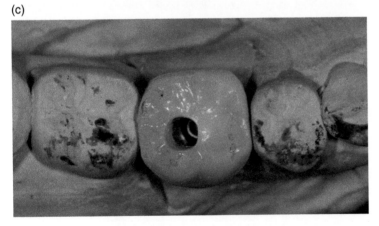

Figure 18.17   (a–f) A suggested protocol for a single implant-supported crown. Contacts should be made according to morphology adopting the conformative approach and a stabilisation splint is used in this patient with bruxism.

(d)

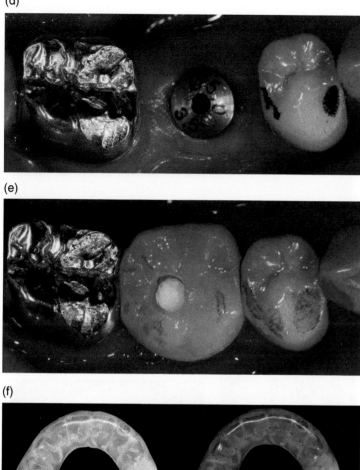

(e)

(f)

Figure 18.17 (Cont'd)

occlusal records of the starting point are extremely helpful. Annual monitoring is recommended.

Suggested Clinical Protocols

Single Implant-Supported Crown

- Implant-supported crowns should contact at 40 µm but there should be no contact at 20 µm.

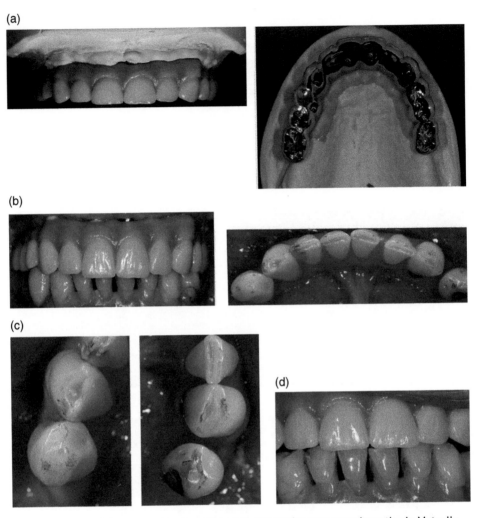

Figure 18.18   (a–d) A suggested protocol for a full arch implant-supported prosthesis. Mutually protected occlusion – anterior guidance shared and disclusion of posterior teeth.

- Contacts should be made according to morphology (conformative approach), avoiding incline contacts.
- Share guidance in parafunctional patients.
- In the lab, a new implant screw is torqued to 25 ncm as per implant system to ensure the same tightening when designing the implant occlusion (Figure 18.17).
- Shared equal centric stops in centric relation
- Group function in lateral guidance with disclusion of non-working side.
- Canine guidance can be provided if implant in canine region is long (riskier).
- Mutually protected occlusion – anterior guidance shared and disclusion of posterior teeth (Figure 18.18).

Further Reading

Davies, S. and Gray, R. (2002). *A Clinical Guide to Occlusion*. London: British Dental Association.

Mish, C. (2014). *Dental Implant Prosthetics*. 2nd Edition. St Louis, MO: Elsevier Mosby.

Resnik, R. (2017). *Principles of Implant Occlusion: Part 2 - Recommendations for Single Implant Prostheses*. Glidewell.

Santos, J.D. (2007). *Occlusion: Principles and Treatment*. London: Quintessence.

Wassell, R., Naru, A., Steele, J., and Nohl, F. (2015). *Applied Occlusion*, 2nd edn. London: Quintessence.

Glossary of Terms

This glossary contains not only terms used in this text but also other terms that the reader might find useful in the field of the masticatory system. Think of this section not so much as a glossary but more as a dictionary.

Abfraction The pathological loss of hard tooth substance caused by biomechanical loading forces.

Angle's classification of occlusion Eponym for a classification system of occlusion based on the interdigitation of the first molar teeth, originally described by Angle as four major groups depending on the anteroposterior jaw relationship.

Anterior guidance Guidance of the mandible during eccentric movements as provided by occlusal contacts. See also Ideal anterior guidance; Posterior guidance.

Articular Of or relating to a joint.

Articular eminence The anterior slope of the glenoid fossa, down which the condyle moves during mouth opening.

Articulate (i) To join together as a joint; (ii) the relating of contacting surfaces of the teeth or their artificial replicas in the maxillae to those in the mandible.

Articulating paper Ink-coated paper strips used to locate and mark occlusal contacts.

Articulating surfaces The fibrous tissue-covered surfaces of both the mandibular condyle and glenoid fossa.

Articulation The place of union or junction between two or more bones of the skeleton. In dentistry, the static and dynamic contact relationship between the occlusal surfaces of the teeth during function.

Articulator A mechanical instrument that represents the temporomandibular joints and jaws, to which maxillary and mandibular casts may be attached to simulate some or all mandibular movements.

Articulatory system Comprises the temporomandibular joints, masticatory muscles, occlusion.

Attrition The act of wearing or grinding down by friction, or mechanical wear resulting from mastication or parafunction, limited to contacting surfaces of the teeth.

Autopolymerising resin A resin, the polymerization of which is initiated by a chemical activator.

Practical Procedures in Dental Occlusion, First Edition. Ziad Al-Ani and Riaz Yar.
© 2022 John Wiley & Sons Ltd. Published 2022 by John Wiley & Sons Ltd.
Companion website: www.wiley.com/go/al-ani-and-riaz/dental-occlusion

Average value articulator An articulator that is fabricated to permit motion based on mean mandibular movements; also called class III articulator.

Axial loading The force directed down the long axis of a body usually used to describe the force of occlusal contact on a natural tooth, dental implant or other object; axial loading is best described as the force down the long axis of the tooth or whatever body is being described.

Balanced articulation The bilateral, simultaneous, anterior and posterior occlusal contact of teeth in centric and eccentric positions.

Balancing side See Non-working side.

Bilateral balanced articulation Also termed balanced articulation, the bilateral, simultaneous anterior and posterior occlusal contact of teeth in centric and eccentric positions.

Bimanual manipulation technique A method for placement of the mandible using both thumbs on the chin and the fingers on the inferior border of the mandible to guide the jaw into centric relation.

Bite See Occlusion.

Bite of convenience See Centric occlusion.

Border movement Mandibular movement at the limits dictated by anatomical structures, as viewed in a given plane.

Bruxism A habitual tooth-grinding activity. See also Parafunction.

Canine guidance An example of an ideal anterior guidance, in which the upper canine exclusively provides the guidance during mandibular lateral excursion.

Canine protected occlusion See Canine guidance.

Centric occlusion (CO) The static tooth relationship into which patients habitually close their teeth.

Centric relation (CR) A reproducible jaw position, independent of tooth contact, which conceptually is the position of the mandible relative to the skull when the muscles are at their most relaxed and least strained position. Anatomically, the disc must be in place and the head of the condyle in its most superior position and in the terminal hinge axis.

Centric relation appliance See Stabilisation splint.

Centric relation occlusion This is the occlusion when the teeth meet evenly without any premature contacts in the centric relation jaw position. See also Centric occlusion; Centric relation.

Centric relation record A registration of the relationship of the maxilla to the mandible when the mandible is in centric relation.

Centric slide The movement of the mandible while in centric relation, from the initial occlusal contact into maximum intercuspation.

Cheek ridging Ridging of the buccal mucosa, usually along the occlusal plane; taken as a sign of active bruxism.

Clenching A habitual contraction of masticatory elevator muscles when the teeth are together and independent of normal function, often resulting in muscle symptoms. See also Parafunction.

Condylar axis A hypothetical line through the mandibular condyles around which the mandible may rotate.

Condylar guidance Mandibular guidance generated by the condyle and articular disc traversing the contour of the glenoid fossae.

Condylar guide assembly The components of an articulator that guide movement of the condylar analogues.

Condylar guide inclination The angle formed by the inclination of a condylar guide control surface of an articulator and a specified reference plane.

Condylar hinge position The position of the condyles of the mandible in the glenoid fossae, at which hinge axis movement is possible.

Condylar inclination The direction of the lateral condyle path.

Condylar path element The member of a dental articulator that controls the direction of condylar movement.

Condyle In the mandible, the projection of bone that articulates with the glenoid fossa.

Craniomandibular articulation Both temporomandibular joints functioning together as a bilateral sliding hinge joint connecting the mandible to the cranium.

Crossover interference A posterior interference when the mandible has reached or exceeded the canine crossover position. See also Posterior interference; Crossover position.

Crossover position The position during lateral mandibular excursion; when in a class I or II occlusion, the mandibular canine is labial to the maxillary canine.

Dahl concept This describes a method of creating interocclusal space in a localised part of the mouth to enable placement of restorations on worn teeth but also has use in a variety of other clinical situations.

Decreased occlusal vertical dimension A reduction in the distance measured between two anatomical points when the teeth are in occlusal contact.

Deflective occlusal contact A contact that displaces a tooth or diverts the mandible from its intended movement. See also Occlusal disharmony; Occlusal prematurity.

Dental panoramic tomogram (DPT) A scanning radiograph showing the dental tissues and associated bones. A modified projection can image the head of condyle.

Deviation of mandibular movement During opening or closing of the mandible, a discursive movement that may be lasting or transient.

Diagnostic cast A life-size reproduction of a part of the oral cavity for the purpose of study and treatment planning.

Diagnostic occlusal adjustment An evaluation of the process and implications of subtractive tooth adjustment on articulator-mounted casts, for determination of the benefits and consequences of an occlusal adjustment.

Direction of slide Direction of mandibular movement when moving from the first contact in centric relation to maximum intercuspation in centric occlusion. See also Centric relation; Centric occlusion; Premature contact.

Dynamic occlusion The contacts between the teeth when the mandible is moving relative to the maxilla.

Dysfunction A collective term for signs and symptoms of an abnormal or altered function.

Earbow An instrument similar to a facebow that indexes the external auditory meatus and registers the relation of the maxillary dental arch to the external auditory meatus and a horizontal reference plane. This instrument is used to transfer the maxillary cast to the articulator. The earbow provides an average anatomical dimension between the external auditory meatus and the horizontal axis of the mandible. See also Facebow.

Eccentric mandibular movement An excursive movement of the mandible relative to the maxilla from centric occlusion.

Equilibration A demanding clinical procedure in which permanent and irreversible changes are made to the patient's natural dentition, with the objective of providing a more ideal occlusion.

Excursive movements See Lateral excursion; Protrusion.

Facebow A device used in mounting the maxillary cast in a semi-adjustable articulator by recording the relationship between the maxillary teeth and the estimated condylar position.

Facebow fork That component of the facebow used to attach the occlusal rim to the facebow.

Facebow record The registration obtained by means of a facebow.

Facebow transfer The process of transferring the facebow record of the spatial relationship of the maxillary arch to some anatomical reference point(s) and transferring this relationship to an articulator.

Facet (wear facet) An area on a tooth or restoration worn down by attrition.

Fossa An anatomical pit, groove or depression.

Fox appliance See Stabilisation splint.

Freedom in centric (long centric) Freedom in centric occlusion occurs when the mandible can move anteriorly for a small distance in the same horizontal and sagittal plane while maintaining tooth contact.

Fully adjustable articulator An articulator that allows replication of three-dimensional movement of recorded mandibular motion – also called a class IV articulator.

Functional mandibular movements All normal, proper or characteristic movements of the mandible made during speech, mastication, yawning, swallowing and other associated movements.

Functional occlusal harmony The occlusal relationship of opposing teeth in all functional ranges and movements that will provide the greatest masticatory efficiency without causing undue strain or trauma on the supporting tissues.

Functional occlusal splint A device that directs the movements of the mandible by controlling the plane and range of motion.

Functional occlusion The contacts of the maxillary and mandibular teeth during mastication and deglutition.

Glenoid fossa The concavity in the temporal bone by the zygomatic arch that receives the mandibular condyle.

Gliding movement See Translation.

Group function An example of an ideal anterior guidance in which usually the maxillary canine, premolar and even buccal cusps of the first molars provide the guidance during lateral excursions of the mandible. The earliest and hardest contacts are provided towards the front of the group.

Guidance Providing regulation or direction to movement; a guide – the influence on mandibular movements by the contacting surfaces of the maxillary and mandibular anterior teeth; mechanical forms on the lower anterior portion of an articulator that guide movements of its upper member. See Anterior guidance; Condylar guidance.

Habitual bite See Centric occlusion.

Hinge axis An imaginary line around which the mandible may rotate within the sagittal plane.

Hyperactivity Excessive motor activity.

Hypertonicity Increased resting muscle activity resulting in an excessive contractile state.

Iatrogenic Resulting from the activity of the clinician; applied to disorders induced in the patient by the clinician.

Ideal anterior guidance Canine guidance or group function with posterior disclusion. See also Ideal occlusion; Anterior guidance; Posterior guidance.

Ideal occlusion A centric occlusion that occurs in centric relation from which excentric movements of the mandible can occur with anterior guidance at the front of the mouth and with posterior disclusion. See also Canine guidance; Centric occlusion; Centric relation; Group function; Ideal anterior guidance; Posterior interference.

Incisal guidance The influence of the contacting surfaces of the mandibular and maxillary anterior teeth on mandibular movements; the influences of the contacting surfaces of the guide pin and guide table on articulator movements.

Incisal guide angle Anatomically, the angle formed by the intersection of the plane of occlusion and a line within the sagittal plane determined by the incisal edges of the maxillary and mandibular central incisors, when the teeth are in maximum intercuspation. On an articulator, that angle formed, in the sagittal plane, between the plane of reference and the slope of the anterior guide table, as viewed in the sagittal plane.

Incisal opening A measurement of mouth opening taken from incisor tip to incisor tip. Usually recorded at both 'pain-free' and 'maximal' opening levels.

Infraocclusion Occlusion in which the occluding surfaces of teeth are below the normal plane of occlusion.

Intercondylar distance The distance between the rotational centres of two condyles or their analogues.

Intercuspal contact The contact between the cusps of opposing teeth.

Intercuspal contact area The range of tooth contacts in maximum intercuspation.

Intercuspation position (ICP) A synonym for centric occlusion.

Interference In dentistry, any tooth contacts that interfere with or hinder harmonious mandibular movement.

Interocclusal Between the occlusal surfaces of opposing teeth.

Interocclusal clearance The arrangement in which the opposing occlusal surfaces may pass each other without any contact; the amount of reduction achieved during tooth preparation to provide for an adequate thickness of restorative material.

Interocclusal distance The distance between the occluding surfaces of the maxillary and mandibular teeth when the mandible is in a specified position.

Interocclusal gap See Interocclusal distance.

Interocclusal record A registration of the positional relationship of the opposing teeth or arches; a record of the positional relationship of the teeth or jaws to each other.

Interocclusal rest space The difference between the vertical dimension at rest and the vertical dimension while in occlusion.

Intracondylar Within the condyle.

Initial occlusal contact During closure of the mandible, the first or initial contact of opposing teeth between the arches.

Jig A device used to maintain mechanically the correct positional relationship between a piece of work and a tool, or between components during assembly or alteration.

Kinematic axis The transverse horizontal axis connecting the rotational centres of the right and left condyles.

Kinematic facebow A facebow with adjustable calliper ends used to locate the transverse horizontal axis of the mandible.

Kinematics The phase of mechanics that deals with the possible motions of a material body.

Lateral condylar inclination The angle formed by the path of the moving condyle within the horizontal plane compared with the median plane (anteroposterior movement) and within the frontal plane when compared with the horizontal plane (superoinferior movement).

Lateral condylar path The path of movement of the condyle–disc assembly in the joint cavity when a lateral mandibular movement is made.

Lateral excursion Movement of the mandible relative to the maxilla, primarily in the right or left lateral direction.

Laterodetrusion Lateral and downward movement of the condyle on the working side.

Lateroprotrusion A protrusive movement of the mandibular condyle in which there is a lateral component.

Lateroretrusion Lateral and backward movement of the condyle on the working side.

Laterosurtrusion Lateral and upward movement of the condyle on the working side.

Laterotrusion Condylar movement on the working side in the horizontal plane. This term may be used in combination with terms describing condylar movement in other planes, e.g. laterodetrusion, lateroprotrusion, lateroretrusion and laterosurtrusion.

Long centric See Freedom in centric.

Lucia jig An individually fabricated anterior guide table that allows mandibular motion without the influence of tooth contacts, and facilitates the recording of maxillomandibular relationships.

Malocclusion Any deviation from a physiologically acceptable contact between the opposing dental arches; any deviation from a normal occlusion.

Mandibular dysfunction See Myofascial pain.

Mandibular hinge position The position of the mandible in relation to the maxilla, at which opening and closing movements occur on the hinge axis.

Masseter muscle A muscle originating from the inferior aspect of the anterior two-thirds of the zygomatic arch and inserting into the lateral aspect of the angle of the mandible. In normal function, one of the principal elevator muscles of the mandible.

Masticating cycles The patterns of mandibular movements formed during the chewing of food.

Mastication The process of chewing food for swallowing and digestion.

Masticatory apparatus See Masticatory system.

Masticatory cycle A three-dimensional representation of mandibular movement produced during the chewing of food.

Masticatory efficiency The effort required in achieving a standard degree of comminution.

Masticatory force The force applied by the muscles of mastication during chewing.

Masticatory movements Mandibular movements used for chewing food. See also Masticatory cycle.

Masticatory muscles Muscles that elevate the mandible to close the mouth (temporalis, superficial and deep masseter, and medial pterygoid).

Masticatory pain Discomfort about the face and mouth induced by chewing or other use of the jaws, but independent of local disease involving the teeth and mouth.

Masticatory performance A measure of the comminution of food attainable under standardised testing conditions.

Masticatory system Comprises the teeth, periodontal tissues and articulatory system.

Maxillomandibular registration See Maxillomandibular relationship record.

Maxillomandibular relationship Any spatial relationship of the maxillae to the mandible; any one of the infinite relationships of the mandible to the maxillae.

Maxillomandibular relationship record A registration of any positional relationship of the mandible relative to the maxillae. These records may be made at any vertical, horizontal or lateral orientation.

Maximal intercuspal contacts Tooth contact in the maximum intercuspal position.

Maximal intercuspal position The complete intercuspation of the opposing teeth independent of condylar position, sometimes referred to as the best fit of the teeth regardless of the condylar position – also called maximal intercuspation. See Centric occlusion.

Meatus A natural body passage; a general term for any opening or passageway in the body.

Medial pterygoid A muscle originating from between the pterygoid plates and inserting into the medial aspect of the angle of the mandible. In normal function, active in closing and excursive movements of the mandible.

Mediotrusion A movement of the condyle medially. See also Non-working side.

Michigan splint See Stabilisation splint.

Microtrauma Minor injury which, if repetitive, may cause damage.

Muscle contraction The shortening and development of tension in a muscle in response to stimulation.

Muscle contracture A condition of high resistance to passive stretching of a muscle, resulting from fibrosis of the tissues supporting the muscle or the joint; sustained increased resistance to passive stretch with reduced muscle length.

Muscle hyperalgesia Increased sensitivity to pain in a muscle evoked by stimulation at the site of pain in the muscle.

Muscle hypertension Increased muscular tension that is not easily released but does not prevent normal lengthening of the muscles involved.

Muscle hypertonicity Increased contractile activity in some motor units driven by reflex arcs from receptors in the muscle and/or α motoneurons of the spinal cord.

Muscle spasm A sudden involuntary contraction of a muscle or group of muscles attended by pain and interference with function. It differs from muscle splinting in that the contraction is sustained even when the muscle is at rest, and the pain/dysfunction is present with passive and active movements of the affected part; also called myospasm.

Muscle spasticity Increased muscular tension of antagonists preventing normal movement and caused by an inability to relax (a loss of reciprocal inhibition).

Muscle tone Resting muscle activity. See also Muscle hypertonicity.

Muscular atrophy A wasting of muscular tissue, especially due to lack of use.

Muscular splinting Contraction of a muscle or group of muscles attended by interference with function and producing involuntary movement and distortion; differs from muscle spasm in that the contraction is not sustained when the muscle is at rest.

Mutually protected articulation An occlusal scheme in which the posterior teeth prevent excessive contact of the anterior teeth in maximum intercuspation, and the anterior teeth disengage the posterior teeth in all mandibular excursive movements. Alternatively, an occlusal scheme in which the anterior teeth disengage the posterior teeth in all mandibular excursive movements, and the posterior teeth prevent excessive contact of the anterior teeth in maximum intercuspation.

Mutually protected occlusion See Mutually protected articulation.

Myofascial trigger point A hyperirritable spot, usually within a skeletal muscle or in the muscle fascia, that is painful on compression and can give rise to characteristic referred pain, tenderness (secondary hyperalgesia) and autonomic phenomena.

Myofunctional Relating to the function of muscles. In dentistry, the role of muscle function in the cause or correction of muscle-related problems.

Myogenous pain Deep somatic musculoskeletal pain originating in skeletal muscles, fascial sheaths or tendons.

Myositis Inflammation of muscle tissue.

Myospasm See Muscle spasm.

Myostatic contracture Muscle contracture resulting from reduced muscle stimulation.

Myotonia Increased muscular irritability and contractility with decreased power of relaxation; tonic muscle spasms.

Neck of the condylar process The constricted inferior portion of the mandibular condylar process that is continuous with the ramus of the mandible; that portion of the condylar process that connects the mandibular ramus to the condyle.

Neuromuscular release A term used by some clinicians to describe a reduction in contractile and electric activity of the masticatory muscles.

Non-working side The side from which the mandible moves during lateral excursion.

Non-working side condyle path The path that the condyle traverses on the non-working side when the mandible moves in lateral excursion, which may be viewed in the three reference planes of the body.

Non-working side interference A posterior occlusal contact on the non-working side, during lateral excursion of the mandible. See also Non-working side.

Noxious stimulus A tissue-damaging stimulus.

Occlude To bring together; to shut; to bring or close the mandibular teeth into contact with the maxillary teeth.

Occlusal Pertaining to the masticatory surfaces of the posterior teeth, prostheses or occlusion rims.

Occlusal adjustment Any change in the occlusion intended to alter the occluding relation; any alteration of the occluding surfaces of the teeth or restorations.

Occlusal contact The touching of opposing teeth on elevation of the mandible – any contact relation of opposing teeth. See also Deflective occlusal contact; Initial occlusal contact.

Occlusal disharmony A phenomenon in which contacts of opposing occlusal surfaces are not in harmony with other tooth contacts and/or the anatomical and physiological components of the craniomandibular complex.

Occlusal force The result of muscular force applied to opposing teeth; the force created by the dynamic action of the muscles during the physiological act of mastication; the result of muscular activity applied to opposing teeth.

Occlusal harmony A condition in centric and eccentric jaw relation in which there are no interceptive or deflective contacts of occluding surfaces.

Occlusal interference Any tooth contact that inhibits the remaining occluding surfaces from achieving stable and harmonious contacts.

Occlusal prematurity Any contact of opposing teeth that occurs before the planned intercuspation.

Occlusal reduction The quantity (usually measured in millimetres) of tooth structure that is removed to establish adequate space for a restorative material between the occlusal aspect of the tooth preparation and the opposing dentition.

Occlusal registration A method of physically recording the contacts between the teeth.

Occlusal splint An intraoral appliance of variable design used in the management of a temporomandibular disorder or parafunction.

Occlusal stability The equalisation of contacts that prevent tooth movement after closure.

Occlusal trauma Trauma to the periodontium from functional or parafunctional forces causing damage to the attachment apparatus of the periodontium by exceeding its adaptive and reparative capacities. It may be self-limiting or progressive.

Occlusal vertical dimension The distance measured between two points when the occluding members are in contact.

Occlusal wear Loss of substance on opposing occlusal units or surfaces as the result of attrition or abrasion.

Occlusion The act or process of closure or of being closed or shut off; the static relationship between the incising or masticating surfaces of the maxillary or mandibular teeth or tooth analogues.

Occlusion analysis A systematic examination of the masticatory system with special consideration of the effect of tooth occlusion on the teeth and their related structures.

Occlusion record A registration of opposing occluding surfaces made at any maxillomandibular relationship.

Panoramic radiograph A tomogram of the maxilla and mandible taken with a specialised machine designed to present a panoramic view of the full circumferential lengths of the maxilla and mandible on a single film; also called orthopantograph.

Panoramic radiography A method of radiography by which a continuous radiograph of the maxillary and/or mandibular dental arches and their associated structures may be obtained.

Parafunction A function carried out to an abnormal degree (e.g. clenching, tooth grinding) during the day or night and of which the person may be unaware.

Passive manipulation A technique for finding the path of closure to centric relation. See also Centric relation.

Pathogenic occlusion An occlusal relationship capable of producing pathological changes in the stomatognathic system.

Physical elasticity of muscle The physical quality of muscle of being elastic, i.e. yielding to active or passive physical stretch.

Physiological elasticity of muscle The unique biological quality of muscle of being capable of change and of resuming its original size under neuromuscular control.

Physiological occlusion Occlusion in harmony with the functions of the masticatory system.

Physiologically balanced occlusion A balanced occlusion that is in harmony with the temporomandibular joints and neuromuscular system.

Plain radiography Aasic two-dimensional imaging using an x-ray source and conventional film/cassettes.

Polyvinyl siloxane A silicone elastomeric impression material of silicone polymers that has terminal vinyl groups that cross-link with silanes on activation by a platinum or palladium salt catalyst.

Posterior guidance Guidance of the mandible during eccentric movements provided by the temporomandibular joint. See also Anterior guidance; Ideal anterior guidance.

Posterior interference Any predominant contact between the back teeth on excentric movements of the mandible.

Premature contact in CR First tooth contact when the mandible is in centric relation.

Protrusion Movement of the mandible relative to the maxilla that is primarily in an anterior direction. See also Lateral protrusion.

Protrusive Thrusting forward; adjective denoting protrusion.

Protrusive condyle path The path that the condyle travels when the mandible is moved forward from its initial position.

Protrusive deflection A continuing excentric displacement of the midline incisal path on protrusion, symptomatic of a restriction of movement.

Protrusive deviation Discursive movement on protrusion that ends in the centred position and is indicative of interference during movement.

Protrusive interocclusal record A registration of the mandible in relation to the maxilla when both condyles are advanced in the temporal fossa.

Protrusive jaw relation A jaw relation resulting from protrusion of the mandible.

Protrusive movement Mandibular movement anterior to centric relation.

Protrusive occlusion An occlusion of the teeth when the mandible is protruded.

Protrusive record See Protrusive interocclusal record.

Protrusive relation The relation of the mandible to the maxillae when the mandible is thrust forward.

Range of motion The range, measured in degrees of a circle, through which a joint can be extended or flexed. The range of the opening, lateral and protrusive excursions of the temporomandibular joint.

Registration The making of a record of the jaw relationships present, or those desired, thus allowing their transfer to an articulator to assist in proper fabrication of a dental prosthesis; a record made of the desired maxillomandibular relationship and used to relate casts to an articulator.

REM period of sleep (rapid eye movement) An active period of sleep usually just before waking, during which there are periods of increased muscle activity.

Remodel The morphological change in bone as an adaptive response to altered environmental demands. The bone will progressively remodel where there is proliferation of tissue and regressive remodelling occurs when osteoclastic resorption is evident.

Retruded contact Contact of a tooth or teeth along the retruded path of closure. Initial contact of a tooth or teeth during closure around a transverse horizontal axis.

Retruded contact position (RCP) A synonym for centric relation.

Semi-adjustable articulator An articulator that permits replication of average mandibular movements.

Shimstock A thin (8–12 μm) strip of polyester film used to identify the presence or absence of occlusal or proximal contacts.

Soft bite guard (soft splint) Resilient polyvinyl vacuum-formed device covering the mandibular teeth made to no particular occlusion for the suggested purpose of preventing trauma to the dentition.

Splint See Occlusal splint.

Stabilisation splint A hard acrylic splint designed to provide an ideal occlusion. Synonyms – Michigan splint, Tanner appliance, Fox appliance, centric relation appliance.

Static occlusion The contacts between the teeth when the mandible is closed in centric occlusion.

Stomatognathic system The combination of structures involved in speech, mastication and deglutition as well as parafunctional actions.

Study cast See Diagnostic cast.

Superior pterygoid The superior head of the lateral pterygoid muscle inserted into the anterior extension of the intra-articular disc. Active in the close/clench cycle. See also Lateral pterygoid.

Tanner appliance See Stabilisation splint.

Temporalis muscle A muscle originating from the temporal fossa, running below the zygomatic arch to insert into the anterior aspect of the coronoid process. In normal function, one of the principal elevator muscles.

Temporomandibular disorders (TMDs) A collective term encompassing conditions that affect the articulatory system.

Temporomandibular joint (TMJ) The articulation of the condylar process of the mandible and the intra-articular disc with the mandibular fossa of the squamous portion of the temporal bone; a diarthrodial sliding and rotating joint. Movement in the upper joint compartment is mostly translational, whereas that in the lower joint compartment is mostly rotational. The joint connects the mandibular condyle to the articular fossa of the temporal bone with the temporomandibular disc interposed.

Temporomandibular joint hypermobility Excessive mobility of the temporomandibular joint.

Terminal hinge axis The axis of closure when the mandible is in centric relation. See also Centric relation.

Tongue habit Conscious or unconscious movements of the tongue that are not related to purposeful functions. Such habits may produce malocclusion or injuries to tissues of the tongue or the attachment apparatus of the teeth.

Tongue scalloping Scalloping of the tongue with characteristic indentations along the lateral border of the tongue; taken as a sign of active bruxism.

Tongue thrusting The infantile pattern of suckle–swallow in which the tongue is placed between the incisor teeth or alveolar ridges during the initial stages of deglutition, resulting sometimes in an anterior open occlusion, deformation of the jaws and/or abnormal function.

Translation That motion of a rigid body in which a straight line passing through any two points always remains parallel to its initial position. The motion may be described as a sliding or gliding motion.

Translatory movement The motion of a body at any instant when all points within the body are moving at the same velocity and in the same direction.

Trigger point Irritable focus in a soft tissue structure, most commonly muscle, which, when stimulated, is locally tender and may give rise to referred pain.

Trismus A reduced ability to open the mouth, due to increased tonic contraction of muscle.

Unstrained jaw relation The relation of the mandible to the skull when a state of balanced tonus exists among all the muscles involved; any jaw relation that is attained without undue or unnatural force and that causes no undue distortion of the tissues of the temporomandibular joints.

Vertical axis of the mandible An imaginary line around which the mandible may rotate through the horizontal plane.

Vertical dimension The distance between two selected anatomical or marked points, one on a fixed (usually the tip of the nose) and one on a movable member (usually the chin).

Vertical dimension decrease Decreasing the vertical distance between the mandible and the maxillae by modifications of teeth, the positions of teeth or occlusion rims, or through alveolar or residual ridge resorption.

Vertical dimension increase Increasing the vertical distance between the mandible and the maxillae by modifications of teeth, the positions of teeth or occlusion rims.

Wear facets See Facet.

Working side The side to which the mandible moves during lateral excursion.

Working side condyle The condyle on the working side.

Working side condyle path The path that the condyle travels on the working side when the mandible moves in a lateral excursion.

Working side contacts Contacts of teeth made on the side of the articulation toward which the mandible is moved during working movements.

Working side interference A posterior occlusal contact on the working side, during lateral excursion of the mandible. See also Working side.

Further Reading

Academy of Prosthodontics (2017). The glossary of prosthodontic terms. *J. Prosthet. Dent.* 55: e1–e105.

Al-Ani, Z. and Gray, R.J.M. (2021). Temporomandibular Disorders: A Problem-Based Approach, 2nd edn. Chichester: John Wiley & Sons Ltd.

Gray, R.J.M., Davies, S., and Quayle, A.A. (1997). A clinical guide to temporomandibular disorders. *Br. Dent. J.* 177: 135–142.

Short Answer Questions

1. A 43-year-old patient presents with a fractured palatal cusp of an upper five after eating a sandwich. On examination, the following were found.
   - Extraoral: large masseters, bitten fingernails.
   - Intraoral: healthy periodontium (no BPE > 1). The palatal cusp of the upper vital and unrestored five is fractured subgingivally. Anterior tooth wear, dentine exposure on both upper canine cusp tips.

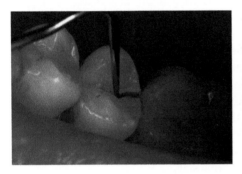 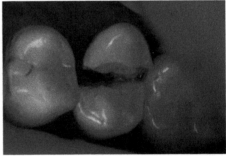

   What is the mechanism leading to this problem?

   What is the significance of the anterior wear?

   What additional precautions might you take in this case when you plan for a definitive restorative work?

2. What is the clinical significance of the last tooth in the arch?

3. What instruments do you need to perform an occlusal examination?

4. Why should thin articulating papers be used in occlusal examination?

5. How should an RCP-ICP slide be assessed?

6. What are the characteristics of good occlusal registration?

7. What should ICP contacts ideally look like?

8. How can fremitus be detected?

Practical Procedures in Dental Occlusion, First Edition. Ziad Al-Ani and Riaz Yar.
© 2022 John Wiley & Sons Ltd. Published 2022 by John Wiley & Sons Ltd.
Companion website: www.wiley.com/go/al-ani-and-riaz/dental-occlusion

9. What are the general occlusal concepts when reorganising the occlusion?

10. What is the custom incisal guide table technique used for?

11. How would you consent a patient for a Dahl concept treatment plan?

12. What are the occlusal factors which might have contributed to the failure of the post crown shown below? What precautions might you take in this case when planning for a new post crown for this patient?

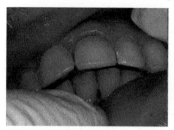 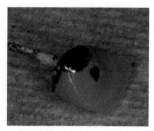 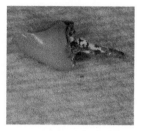

13. Why is the freedom in centric concept particularly important in implant dentistry?

14. What methods can be used to ensure the accuracy of articulated models in the laboratory?

15. Describe the characteristics of a well-balanced stabilisation splint (see illustration below).

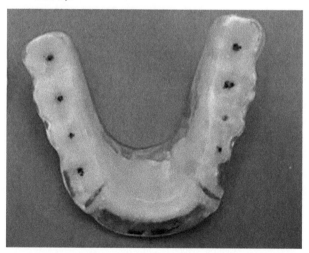

16. What are the differences between average value articulators and semi-adjustable articulators?

17. Properly articulated models mounted with the use of a facebow are essential when a bridge includes occlusal surfaces involved in guidance. Discuss.

18. STOP is a protocol used in this book to be followed for an occlusal practice. What does it stand for?

19. The restorability assessment is important before delivering a restoration because patients' expectations need to be managed. What would you assess?

20. How can we establish canine guidance using a direct composite technique?

Index

Practical Procedures in Dental Occlusion, First Edition. Ziad Al-Ani and Riaz Yar.
© 2022 John Wiley & Sons Ltd. Published 2022 by John Wiley & Sons Ltd.
Companion website: www.wiley.com/go/al-ani-and-riaz/dental-occlusion